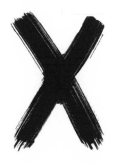

X-OUT CANCER
WITH EXERCISE

EXERCISE HANDBOOK FOR
CANCER PREVENTION & RECOVERY

MANDY ROBERTSON, MD

Print ISBN 978-1-54397-038-8

eBook ISBN 978-1-54397-039-5

PREFACE

This book was written with the intent of helping people to use exercise to prevent cancer and improve their recovery from cancer. I have spent decades caring for people as a Doctor of Medicine. My specialty as a Medical Oncologist has allowed me to focus on people afflicted by cancer. I am a life-long athlete who has personally suffered injuries and setbacks similar to others. My desire for this book is to teach you the knowledge I have gained as a Doctor of Medicine and a life-long athlete, to empower you to get and remain well, and cancer free. As a doctor, I regularly say the things in this book during office visits and lectures to cancer survivors who I have been honored to care for over the years, their family members and friends, as well as community members I have encountered. There are many things that need to be considered when exercising to prevent or recover from cancer. I decided that having a summary of all of this important information in one place as a reference would be beneficial for all the people who constantly ask me, 'what can I do to prevent cancer?' Or 'what can I do to recover faster from cancer treatments?' This summary became what I consider a handbook for exercise for the prevention of cancer and recovery from cancer. This not only could benefit everyone who has had cancer, but also those living with cancer, recovering from cancer, or caring for someone with cancer, and importantly also those wanting to prevent cancer all together.

This handbook is not to be considered a prescription. It should not replace your healthcare providers' recommendations to you about exercise and activities specific for you. Healthcare providers individualize their recommendations to their patients' health and healthcare needs. It will not be able to be all inclusive since there are constantly changes in research regarding benefits of exercise for health and wellbeing as well as benefits in preventing and overcoming cancer. It is a tool in your toolbox of tips and tricks to keep yourself healthy. Even if you have not regularly done any physical activity, you can benefit from this book by learning some techniques to help yourself and others. I hope you use this information to feel better, live happy and healthy, and share the skills you learn with those around you.

I try to practice what I teach. By exercising daily, I can prove to others that it is possible to achieve their goals by staying active. You too can mentor healthy behaviors and share those benefits with others. What is presented in this book is attainable. You CAN exercise and improve your health and well-being. You CAN be a mentor to those around you.

I would like to thank my family and friends for supporting me in this effort. Their continued support while I wrote this book is indescribable. They demonstrated the exercises to show limitations people may have and served as the models for the pictures to show all different ages of people CAN perform these exercises. Time is so precious, yet they gave me the time to complete this project even while also continuing my practice as a full time Medical Oncologist. They honestly reviewed my book with valuable feedback. My family encourages me daily to stay healthy which includes daily exercise, stretching, and meditation. I hope my daily exercise routine rubs off on them too so that they may be happy, healthy, and cancer free.

Live by example.

INTRODUCTION

What exactly is exercise and why is it so important? Exercise is the physical effort to improve health. If we consider that sentence further, it is using your body to make your physical and/or mental condition better. Exercise may encompass many different types of activities that can improve health in various ways. This is important because a healthy body can fight and recover from cancer, as well as other illnesses.

Since everyone's ability to move their body is different, this book will give suggestions for those with various abilities, women and men, young and old. In addition, people have various resources for exercising. This book will give a guide no matter what equipment, time, or extra money is available to spend on exercise.

The first section will explain how exercise can help keep you and others well. It delves into the science of what happens when we exercise, how the body responds to exercise, and the interrelationships between exercise and wellness. The next section will give helpful information about how to approach exercise successfully. It will help you know how to prepare, especially if you have limitations, and how to stay on course for getting the most out of your exercise. The third section of this book will give specific types of exercises you can do, including a written explanation and pictorial demonstrations of the exercises. By reviewing all of these exercises, you can come up with your own exercise plan which you can outline in your own journal at the end of the book. To help you put your plan together, I included example exercise plans for people who have had cancer or wish to prevent cancer. These example exercise plans tackle specific cancer survivors and some of their potential limitations from treatments they have been through or are going through for their cancer. I mention general precautions to consider when exercising in the second section, and more detailed precautions for specific cancers and treatment side effects in the fourth section. There are so many different types of cancers that it would not be feasible to give an exercise example plan for all the different types of cancers and stages of treatment. I have therefore included the most common cancers and some of the more complicated situations cancer survivors may encounter, as well as frequently encountered examples.

There is a daily journal at the end of the book to document your own plan, successes and failures. With exercise, there really is not failure, but sometimes a lack of reaching the planned goals at the set time point. By documenting where you are in an exercise routine, you can better anticipate potential setbacks and restructure your plan to maintain success. This book will give you the information you need to be prepared in advance, and hopefully avoid too many setbacks. Finally, use this exercise handbook to refer back to regularly as a guide, or when you need encouragement to get or stay active, or when you need a new plan to keep your motivation up, or when you need to support others in their exercise plan. Keep it visible as a daily reminder that you have the power to fight cancer by exercising!

SECTION 1

HOW EXERCISE PLAYS A ROLE IN WELLNESS

CHAPTER 1
WHY BOTHER TO EXERCISE

The lack of exercise can increase the risk of getting cancer. For those who have had cancer, the lack of exercise can increase the risk of recurrence. We are all at risk of cancer, not to mention other health diseases and disorders related to the lack of exercise. We are not only at risk, but so are our family members, friends, neighbors, coworkers, bosses, advisors, assistants, and others who we rely on in our daily lives. The carnage cancer leaves behind can be devastating for all of those affected. When you stop and think about it, we are all affected by cancer in some way whether we are the ones dealing with it or helping someone with cancer, living with someone with cancer, working with or for someone with cancer, and so on. And, we are ALL at risk of getting cancer, no matter our race, sex, age, religion, profession, socioeconomic class.

Recent 2017 statistics in the United States predict 1 in every 2 men and 1 in every 3 women will be diagnosed with cancer in their lifetime. Surprisingly, these rates of cancer development are only slightly higher than 50 years previous to this. These statistics are even more remarkable since they do not include common, non-melanoma skin cancers such as squamous cell and basal cell cancers. Unless otherwise stated, when discussing cancer in this book, it will not include common, non-melanoma skin cancers since generally they are unlikely to be lethal and tend to be relatively slow growing.

Although currently more than 70% of those diagnosed with cancer are cured in the United States, almost 30% are not cured. For those nearly 30% living with cancer and for those who are still dealing with the effects of cancer treatments, there are daily struggles that may change the way they live. Many cancers require surgery which can leave scars, loss of limb, weight loss or weight gain, or change in bowel or bladder function. Other types of cancer treatments can leave other disabilities, some of which can also be permanent such as scarring from radiation and neuropathy from chemotherapy to name a few. For those people living with cancer, they are often on continuous treatments with side effects they must manage on a daily basis. Exercise can improve the many different side effects from the cancer and cancer treatments. Exercise can help people to lose weight or gain weight if needed. Exercise can lead to better functioning of the body and overall better quality of life.

Not only can exercise improve the side effects of cancer and cancer treatments for those who have been affected by cancer, but exercise can also help prevent cancer. Some studies have reported up to about 35% benefit at lowering the risk of cancers by exercising regularly. That means 1 in 3 people may be able to prevent cancer by exercising! Colon cancer is probably the best studied cancer with regards to lowering the risk by exercise. Up to 1 out of every 4 people may be able to lower their risk of colon cancer by exercising regularly. And since colon cancer is currently the second most common cancer in both women and men occurring in about 1 in 23 people, this could significantly reduce the rate of cancers in general. Looking closer at these statistics, if 1 out of every 4 people are able to prevent colon cancer by exercising regularly, then the risk of colon cancer could be decreased from 1 out of every 23 to 1 out of every 30 people. The risk of breast cancer can be reduced by about 1 in 8 with exercising regularly. Endometrial cancer rates can be lowered by about 1 in 5 by regular exercise. The role of regular exercise in preventing other cancers is clear but the amount of benefit is not as well defined. So let's consider the number of people who may be spared the ravages of cancer by regular exercise. If regular exercise can decrease the risk of a cancer by a third, and considering the average number of people who were diagnosed with cancer in 2018 was 1.7 million people, then about 560,000 people would be spared a cancer diagnosis. And with the rising cost of healthcare, a conservative estimate of United States, US, healthcare spending on cancer care in 2018 is 150 billion dollars which would be a cost savings of about 50 billion dollars per year if a third of cancers could be prevented with regular exercise. If we think about the average person's savings, it can save a person with insurance at least $5000 out of pocket expenses per year for treatment of a cancer, not including the loss of money from inability to work.

Exercise can also lower the rates of other health disorders such as diabetes, high cholesterol, hypertension, heart disease, and stroke. This could save even more healthcare dollars and more money in your own pocket. Other benefits of exercise include lowering pain associated with cancer and arthritis, reducing the levels of depression and anxiety, and improving fatigue. Breathing can also be enhanced by exercise. Regular exercise has been shown to reduce the rate of type II diabetes by about 50%. In addition, regular exercise can lower the risk of stroke by about 25% and lower heart disease by about 15%. Research has shown that not only are average people at risk for these common health problems, but cancer survivors are at even higher risk for these and other health problems which can be improved through exercise.

When people have fewer medical problems and feel better, they require fewer medicines and doctor visits which can also be a financial benefit. This allows for less time away from work or school. There has actually been research that shows about an average of $100 per month saved when you exercise regularly even without a cancer diagnosis. So not only can exercise lower your chances of getting cancer, improve your ability to recover from cancer and cancer treatments, and live longer and healthier if you are living with cancer, but many other health and financial benefits can occur with regular exercise.

CHAPTER 2
WHO BENEFITS FROM EXERCISE

Everyone can get benefits from exercise and every type of exercise is beneficial! Yes, it is true. Let's consider this in more detail. Remember, exercise is using your body to improve your physical or mental condition. Most of us think about exercise as only the activities that increase our heart rate and breathing, speed up metabolism and make us sweat, like walking or running. But there are other forms of exercise like meditation that focus on breathing and slowing down the heart rate. These types of non-traditional exercises are also beneficial to our well-being. Incorporating a mixture of the various types of exercises into a routine can help promote different types of healthy living, all of which can benefit us.

Studies have shown that there are increased rates of cancer associated with sedentary lifestyles and obesity. Obesity is currently best correlated with body mass index, BMI. Even though BMI is not a direct measure of body fat, it has been compared to other methods of measuring body fat directly and has been found to be a representative measurement of body fat. Since it is a relatively easy and inexpensive way to estimate body fatness and is comparable to more direct measurements, it is utilized for making generalizable recommendations by major health organizations worldwide. So how can someone figure out what their BMI is currently and what it should be?

You can calculate BMI fairly simply. BMI is a person's weight in kilograms divided by the square of height in meters. Approximately 2.2 pounds is equal to 1 kilogram, and 1 meter is equal to 39.4 inches. By using this information, you can figure out your own BMI. A normal BMI is currently defined between 18 and 25, varying slightly for different populations and countries. Overweight is when BMI is over 25 but less than 30, and obesity is when BMI is over 30. Current statistics report that more than 60% of adults are either overweight or obese in the US with more than 30% considered obese. These figures are also true when looking at current international rates of obesity.

Here is an example of calculating BMI for a 180 pound 6 foot tall man. If 1 kilogram is equal to 2.2 pounds, then 180 pounds divided by 2.2 pounds is approximately 81.8 kilograms. There are 12 inches in a foot, so multiple 12 inches by 6 feet to get his height in inches: 72 inches. To change the inches to meters, remember that one meter is equal to 39.4 inches. So divide his height of 72 inches by 39.4 inches to get approximately 1.83 meters, which then is squared (multiply 1.83 by 1.83) to get 3.34 meters. We now have his weight in kilograms, 81.8, and height in meters, 3.34. Then, BMI is calculated by dividing weight in kilograms by squared height in meters: 81.8 kilogram divided by 3.34 meters equals a BMI of 24. You can use your own weight and height to calculate your own BMI.

It seems shocking that only 20% of adults in the U.S. are meeting the minimum amount of exercise recommended by government health agencies. That means 80% of the US adult population could improve their physical activity rates! These averages have only changed slightly in the last few decades. However, other measures of activity have changed significantly during this time. There is more automobile use for travel rather than walking or biking. There are more sedentary activities done on a regular basis like watching television and using computers. There are more technologically advanced assistive devices to help do regular chores like riding lawn mowers and electric vacuums. There is less activity promoted in school age children including less physical education and recess time. All these things add up to a less active, overweight population.

Regular exercise has been shown to significantly lower the rates of obesity which in turn can lead to lowering the rates of cancers including breast cancer, prostate cancer, colorectal cancer, uterine cancer, ovarian cancer, gastrointestinal cancer, and kidney cancer to name a few. Many of these cancers lead the list of the most common cancers in both women and men. The Continuous Update Project is an ongoing program analyzing global research on how physical activity and weight can affect the risk of cancer and cancer survival. There are currently over 9,000 publications in the database which is used by researchers worldwide. Studies compiled and available for review in this database have shown similar results of increased rates of cancer associated with obesity and sedentary lifestyles no matter the age, race, ethnicity, socioeconomic status or sex. This is becoming true across the world, not just in the US.

Exercise can benefit everyone, including people who have never had cancer, by preventing cancer before it ever has a chance to occur. For those diagnosed with cancer or recovering from cancer treatments, exercise can improve how the treatments are tolerated and help lower the rate of recurrence of cancer. For those living with cancer, exercise can prevent and control other diseases and help make the chronic treatments for cancer better tolerated over time. There are a number of research studies that have proven better survival rates from cancer and lower recurrence rates of cancer in those who exercise on a regular basis. In people who are undergoing treatments for cancer, exercise has been shown in research trials to improve the tolerability and recovery from treatments including surgery, radiation, chemotherapy, and hormonal therapies. For those people who do exercise on a regular basis, they often require fewer medicines, have more energy and have less pain. When recovery from cancer and the treatments for cancer occur more quickly, people can return to a more normal life sooner.

Even though this book was written for adults, it is important to consider how our children are being affected by decreasing activity levels and increasing obesity rates. These higher rates of obesity are now seen in 20% of children. Children who are obese are three times more likely to be obese adults. Only 30% of high school kids are meeting the minimum recommended daily levels of exercise. That means 70% of high school kids need more exercise! There is research starting to show that there may be a link between childhood obesity and childhood cancers, similar to the link between adult obesity and cancers. There is also a link between childhood obesity and other disorders such as diabetes. If obesity continues into adulthood, then the risks of cancer are greater for those individuals who remain obese.

Children learn from and mirror their families, peers, and mentors which includes all of us! But we adults also learn from and mirror our families, peers and mentors. So by exercising, you have the ability to improve not only your personal odds at avoiding, recovering from, or surviving cancer, but also improve the odds of all those around you since you are a peer, mentor, family and friend to many others.

Live by example!

CHAPTER 3
WHAT ARE THE BENEFITS OF EXERCISE

We have already discussed that exercise lowers the risk of cancer and lowers the risk of recurrences, but there are a lot of other health benefits. Exercise can lower the rates of diabetes, high cholesterol, hypertension, heart disease, and stroke. Exercise can improve quality of life by lowering arthritis pain and stiffness, giving a sense of well-being, lowering depression and anxiety, and elevating energy levels which can lessen fatigue. Breathing can also be enhanced by exercise. By improving health through exercise, there can be financial benefits as many people require fewer medications, potentially fewer healthcare visits, fewer medical bills and less time off from work for illness.

When you understand how you are helping yourself be well with each of the exercises you are doing, it encourages you to continue these beneficial activities. This is another part of your success: understanding the science behind how exercise can help you to wellness. The field of medicine called exercise physiology is devoted to the science of how exercise improves health. I will touch on a few of the larger concepts to think about as you get started with your exercise program. There is a lot of published data on exercise physiology you could explore further if more specific information is needed.

When you exercise, chemicals produced in the brain, called neurochemicals, are released including norepinephrine and serotonin. These neurochemicals send messages to your nervous system. Low levels of serotonin are associated with depression and anxiety. Serotonin is increased with exercise. Increased serotonin levels can provide a sense of wellbeing, improving depression and anxiety. Positive emotions have been linked to protective effects on health including lowering mortality from heart disease. Low levels of serotonin can lead to insomnia and poor sleep. By exercising and thereby increasing serotonin levels, depression, anxiety and sleep can all be improved. Norepinephrine, which is another neurochemical released by the brain with exercise, increases heart rate and circulation to muscles, helps the mind to focus, and also improves mood. There are other hormones released during exercise too. These include testosterone, growth hormone, thyroid hormone, epinephrine and insulin. These hormones are involved in strengthening muscles and joints, managing the body's metabolism, and maintaining appropriate weight. Together, the hormones produced during exercise promote healing and improve the functioning of the body.

Endorphins are also increased in the blood of people who participate in vigorous exercise, but how they play a role is not as well understood. Endorphins are structurally similar to morphine and can activate opioid receptors in the brain and elsewhere to minimize pain. This may be how exercise improves arthritis-related pain and the pain associated with scar tissue from surgery or radiation. But the exact mechanism of how the endorphins work at modulating pain is still being researched.

Exercise can improve and prevent pain in other ways as well. By strengthening the muscles that support the joints through exercise, less stress is put on the joints. By less stress put on joints, the pain in those joints is less likely to occur or be as severe. When muscles are stronger and joints are healthier, the risk of fracture is reduced. Also, exercise helps improve coordination and flexibility of the body which can lower the risk of falls. The strengthening of the muscles to support the joints, improved coordination and flexibility all lead to better body mechanics which can promote health, lower injuries, and improve and prevent pain.

There are other important hormones that have been discovered called insulin-like growth factors. High circulating levels of insulin-like growth factor have been associated with increased risks of cancer and worse outcomes from cancer. Insulin-like growth factors are important regulators of cellular growth and turnover. When they don't function normally, it can lead to development of cancers. In addition, cancer cells can use insulin-like growth factor pathways to stimulate replication and grow. Exercise has been shown to decrease the amount of circulating insulin-like growth factors. This in turn may lead to lower rates of cancer development and slower growth of cancers that are already present. Hence, another way exercise can prevent cancer and improve survival of those living with cancer.

During exercise, the tissues of the body use oxygen for energy called cellular metabolism and produce increased amounts of carbon dioxide. The higher levels of carbon dioxide signal the medulla in the brain to increase the rate of breathing. This leads to an increased respiratory rate which then increases oxygen to the blood vessels that supply the tissues of the body. Muscles and organs that are in better shape from regular exercise utilize oxygen more efficiently. This allows the body to require less energy and less oxygen. This is why exercise is important for people who have had heart attacks and have lung diseases like emphysema. Even though their organs have permanent damage, exercise can improve the ability of the organs to more efficiently use oxygen which is necessary for energy as part of daily functioning. The benefit of efficiently using oxygen for the production of energy may also help tissues, organs and cells recover faster from cancer and treatments for cancer, too. Therefore, exercise improves the body's ability to oxygenate itself and provide energy to promote healing and wellness.

Our heart is the main pump system for moving blood around our body. Our lungs are the main location for exchanging oxygen for carbon dioxide. Oxygen is needed for the body's energy and the carbon dioxide is the byproduct that the body produces as it makes energy. Oxygen is absorbed in the lungs as we breathe in air. In the blood vessels that flow through the lungs, carbon dioxide is exchanged for the oxygen which is then carried by the blood in these blood vessels to the tissues and organs of the body where it can be used for energy. It is in the blood vessels of the lungs, some of which are very small, where the transfer of carbon dioxide for oxygen occurs. The red blood cells carry oxygen from the lungs to the tissues of the body for energy where the oxygen is converted to carbon dioxide, a by-product of energy use produced by the tissues of the body. The red blood cells collect the carbon dioxide and deliver it back to the lungs to repeat the process of oxygen exchange. The heart rate increases during exercise in response to the need of more oxygen by the tissues. The heart is also a muscle which requires oxygen to function. Limitations to exercise can occur when people have blood vessel disorders where plaque or other problems narrow the blood vessels, such as in coronary artery disease and peripheral vascular disease. In these types of conditions, the increased oxygen demands of the body from exercise can lead to worse oxygenation of the tissues if the blood cannot circulate through the blood vessels well enough to get to the organs that need extra oxygen. In these conditions, exercise is still important to improve the energy efficiency of the muscles, but a more controlled and gentle exercise program is needed to avoid complications. Therefore, it is always important to check with your healthcare provider when you start a more vigorous exercise program, especially if you have had heart or blood vessel disorders.

Some types of cancer and treatments for cancer can lead to low red blood cell counts called anemia that then limit the amount of oxygen that can be carried through the body. This can affect the ability to do exercises, and leads to inefficiency of the muscles and organs. In addition, cancer surgeries and cancer treatment side effects can limit the ability to absorb oxygen and can also limit oxygen delivery to the tissues. Modification to exercise programs can still allow for participation on a regular basis during these types of conditions. Even when side effects of cancer or cancer treatments cause problems that limit activities and exercise, it is still important to stay as active as possible to prevent muscle weakness, and to stimulate the production of hormones that have been discussed which promotes healing and well-being.

SECTION 2
LET'S GET GOING!

CHAPTER 4
PREPARING TO EXERCISE

It is important to know what limitations you have prior to starting an exercise program so that you have an appropriate plan in place for success. Prior to starting an exercise program, discuss your plan with your healthcare provider to make sure there are no restrictions of exercises you should do based on your personal medical history. For instance, after surgery there is usually a lifting restriction for a limited time. Also, radiation can sometimes cause drying of the skin. In this instance, limiting or avoiding excessive water exposure, which may occur during swimming, might be recommended. If you use oxygen, you may need to also use it or increase what you use during exercises. If you have cardiovascular disease, check with your family healthcare provider or cardiologist to make sure you know what limitations they may have for you, or if you need clearance with certain tests before you begin an exercise routine. Some people with pulmonary or cardiovascular disease may benefit from a rehabilitation program called cardiopulmonary rehab prior to starting a routine exercise program on their own. This is a monitored exercise program where your heart and breathing can be closely monitored while you exercise until you are ready to exercise without the monitoring. Your healthcare provider can help determine if this might benefit you.

Pain can sometimes occur during exercise and should not be ignored. If while you are exercising you have pain, you should stop and consider checking with your healthcare provider before continuing. If you have chest pain or a rapid heart rate that does not slow down when you stop exercising, you should consider calling emergency services or go to the emergency room. It is very uncommon to have major cardiovascular events during exercise, but sometimes there are warning signs of a possible future cardiovascular event. These warning signs can be chest pain or a very rapid heart rate that goes away after you stop exercising. These warning signs should be discussed with your healthcare provider before restarting your exercise program. Other pain, such as knee pain or back pain may mean that you are overusing those areas, or doing the exercise incorrectly. Start slow for short increments and then build up to your ultimate goal. It is as important to rest muscle groups as it is to exercise them, which is why varying exercises and activities is good practice. If the pain persists more than a day or two, you should see a healthcare provider.

Maximizing your cardiovascular benefits during your exercise program can also help you be successful with your plan. When you exercise, there are some basic evaluations that you can do to know if you are reaching and maintaining a good heart rate. Simple things like talking full sentences during exercise will keep you from overdoing it. It is important to know your baseline heart rate at rest. A normal heart rate is between 60-100 beats per minute, bpm, although some people will have a heart rate slightly below 60 bpm. To figure out your maximum heart rate, subtract your age from 220. For instance, a 50 year old will have a maximum heart rate of 170 bpm. To calculate your target heart rate during exercise, multiply your maximum heart rate by 0.5 and by 0.85 which will give you the target range of 50-85% of your maximum heart rate. So a 50 year old will have a target heart rate range of 85-145 bpm during exercise which is 50-85% of their maximum heart rate, 170. Fat burning typically happens at 60-70% of your maximum heart rate, which can be calculated by multiplying your maximum heart rate by 0.6 and 0.7 to get a fat burning range. Usually you will need to reach your fat burning heart rate range for at least 15 minutes to lose weight. Some medicines do not allow your heart rate to increase normally with exercise. This can be confusing if you are trying to reach a particular target range. Check with your healthcare provider to see if you are on a medicine that may alter your heart rate.

There are some other considerations to stay healthy while you exercise. Make sure you dress appropriately for the weather and activity planned. If it is cold outside, wear long pants and long sleeves and consider whether you need gloves and a hat. If you are walking, have good safe walking shoes. Use sunscreen if you are outside even on cloudy days. Think about bug spray if you are in an area at risk of mosquitoes or ticks. Also, stay hydrated. Even when you do not sweat, you lose water through your skin. You should try to drink plenty of non-alcoholic fluids through the day to be hydrated before and after you work out. Try to drink 16 ounces of water an hour to two hours before you exercise, and then 8 ounces prior to exercise and about every 15 minutes during your exercise routine and again after you exercise.

Being prepared for your exercise plan, knowing your limitations before you make your plan, and partnering with your healthcare providers will help you be successful. By discussing your exercise plan with your healthcare provider, you can know in advance any limitations they need you to be aware of for safety. If you experience pain, stop and check with your healthcare provider before continuing with your exercise program. If the pain does not go away after a day or two, or if you have chest pain or palpitations during exercise, you should see your healthcare provider before restarting your exercise program. If your chest pain or palpitations does not go away when you stop your activity, you should seek emergency medical assistance. Finally, dress and prepare appropriately for your activity planned and hydrate well prior to, during and after exercise.

CHAPTER 5
PRECAUTIONS TO CONSIDER

After you have prepared for your exercise program, there are some other common precautions to consider that may occur during your exercise program. There are some signs and symptoms you should watch out for when you are exercising, and certainly not ignore. When you have cancer or are undergoing treatments, there may be additional precautions you would otherwise not think about.

If you feel overly tired during exercise, shorten the time you engage in the activities. You could do a couple short intervals of activity in a day instead of a long interval. Often when you first begin an exercise program or when you are undergoing treatments for cancer, you may not have the energy to complete your exercise all at one time. By splitting your exercise program during the day into smaller sections, your benefits will be similar and you will be more likely to complete it.

Pain can sometimes occur during exercise and should not be ignored. If while you are exercising you have pain, you should stop. If you have chest pain or a rapid heart rate that does not slow down when you stop exercising, you should consider calling emergency services or go to the emergency room. It is very uncommon to have major cardiovascular events during exercise, but sometimes there are warning signs of a possible future cardiovascular event. These warning signs can be chest pain or a very rapid heart rate that goes away when you stop exercising. These warning signs should be discussed with your healthcare provider before restarting your exercise program. Other pain, such as knee pain or back pain may mean that you are overusing those areas, or doing the exercise incorrectly. Start slow for short increments and then build up to your ultimate goal. By resting muscle groups periodically by varying exercises and activities, you will be less likely to have an injury or overuse your muscles. If the pain persists more than a day or two, you should consider seeing a healthcare provider.

There are some limitations of exercise and activities set by your healthcare providers. For instance, after surgery there is usually a lifting restriction for a limited time. There can also be stretching restrictions. Radiation can dry the skin which can limit certain exercises such as swimming or excessive sweating. With chemotherapy treatments, side effects can limit your exercise tolerance or put you at risk for infections which may limit where you exercise. Your healthcare providers can direct you on how to safely exercise depending on the chemotherapy you receive.

Medicines you take can affect your ability to exercise. Certain medicines can cause your heart rate to not increase as you would expect or can lower your blood pressure during exercise. Other medicines may increase your blood pressure and heart rate faster than you expect. If you are on blood thinners, watch for bleeding and be careful of activities that put you at risk for falls. Knowing how your medicines may affect you as you exercise is important to consider.

During cancer treatments or shortly after treatment for cancer, there are additional conditions to be aware of and know about which may affect your exercise plan. Anemia is a low red blood count. If you have anemia, you may need to limit or modify the exercises that you do since your oxygen carrying capacity will be more limited. This can lead to more fatigue, shortness of breath with activities, and sometimes pain. If you have a low white blood cell count, it can put you at risk for infections. Therefore, you may need to modify where you exercise. During times of lowered immune system, you may need to avoid gyms or large crowded areas. If you have skin breakdown or open sores from surgery or radiation treatment, you need to avoid soaking in water, chlorinated water, excessive sun exposure, and excessive sweating. If you have diarrhea or nausea and vomiting from treatments, you may need to minimize or shorten exercise to avoid further dehydration and electrolyte abnormalities. If you are having fevers, you should consider skipping exercises until the fevers are gone. Usually these concerns about treatment-related risks resolve about 3 to 6 months after completion of treatment.

Sometimes cancer survivors have added devices to consider during exercise. If you have feeding tubes, urinary catheters, ostomy bags, or intravenous catheters, it is important to avoid pools, hot tubs, lakes, ocean water or other excessive water exposures that could put you at risk for infection. If the device is covered properly, you may be able to have short exposures to water such as showering. It is important to talk to your healthcare providers about these types of situations. In addition, types of exercises you do with these devices may need to be altered to avoid excessive straining of the muscles near the device to avoid dislodging it, or in the case of an ostomy bag, causing a hernia. It is still important for you to exercise regularly even if you have one of these devices.

If you already have a hernia, then you need to consider this in the development of your exercise plan. A hernia is when the abdominal muscle has become weak in an area and the bowel can slip into that space. If you have a hernia, you should consider wearing a special belt or a tight undergarment, like spandex shorts, to prevent causing the hernia from becoming bigger. Avoiding certain types of abdominal exercises and heavy lifting can help prevent hernias from enlarging as well. If you have sudden pain at the site of a hernia that does not go away within a few minutes, then you need to seek medical attention to make sure the bowel has not become stuck in that space, also called a bowel obstruction. Sometimes hernias become large enough they have to be surgically repaired; talk to your healthcare provider about this if you are concerned about your hernia.

If you have weak bones or cancer affecting your bones, you are at a higher risk of bone fractures. In these instances, you will need to consider activities that do not put a lot of force on the bones and will not put you at risk of falls. Be careful about exercising on uneven surfaces, slippery surfaces, and dark conditions. Use lighter weights with more repetitions rather than heavy weights. Consider stationary exercise machines like reclining bicycles and treadmills, although it is still safe to walk outside during daylight hours on flat surfaces. Exercise can actually help to strengthen bones over time, so it is still important to exercise even if you do have weak bones or if cancer affected your bones.

Overall, exercising is safe and healthy, but you should be aware of any potential limitations and risks that you may have to avoid injury. During exercising, if signs or symptoms come on that are concerning, you should stop and consider seeking medical attention if warranted. Setting goals is important, but modifying your goals to remain healthy is sometimes necessary as well.

CHAPTER 6
HOW TO BE SUCCESSFUL

To be successful with your exercise plan, it is important to do exercises and activities you will enjoy and make it as convenient as possible. If exercise is fun, you will want to do it more often, not avoid it all together. You can incorporate exercise into your daily routine to simplify the day. Staying active is what is important, not just exercise. Studies have shown health benefits with walking, swimming, biking, stretching, yoga, weight-lifting, even just deep breathing exercises. Know that all types of exercises and activities can count towards your total goal each week. Also, doing different exercises not only prevents overuse of muscle groups and injuries, but also prevents boredom from monotonous programs. If you develop some routines into your day of when you exercise, then your exercise goals will be more attainable.

How you reach you exercise time goals each week can be varied. If you are over the age of 20 years old, your goal should be at least 15 to 30 minutes per day of exercise but try to incorporate at least moderate activity such as brisk walking on 3 of the days per week. Brisk walking can be walking at a pace of a mile in about 20 minutes. The total time per day can be split up into smaller increments to be more successful at reaching the total goal. For instance, 10 minutes of walking in the morning, 10 minutes at lunch and 10 minutes at the end of your day gets you 30 minutes total which is the minimum goal per day.

Each person may have a different way of successfully getting their daily exercise accomplished. If you plan ahead to set aside time every day for exercise, you are more likely to complete it. Try to do some of your exercises in the morning to help start your day off better physically and prevent not doing the exercise altogether. Make it part of your daily routine to be more successful. Here are some examples of easy ways to incorporate exercise into your day. Park further away from your destination than you would normally park to add a short walk. Instead of taking the short route to your mailbox, walk around the block to get your mail. Park at the back of the store parking lot to add distance to your walk. Volunteer to walk your neighbor's dog. Walk during your kids activities like sports practices. Do some exercises while you watch television. At work you can incorporate activities which will count like taking the stairs instead of the elevator, or at lunchtime incorporating a walk, time to stretch, or do some deep breathing exercises. You could walk or bike to work and home. Each person will have different schedules to fit in various activities efficiently to their daily schedule to get to their desired total time accrued per week.

Remind yourself regularly of your goals and successes. Write yourself a reminder or positive reaffirmation of your goals for the day such as with a crayon on your bathroom mirror, with chalk on your front or back porch, or on paper on your fridge. Put it somewhere you see regularly to remind yourself of your plan and your successes. Positive reinforcement helps you as much as others who see your successes and your determination.

It is easy to lose steam and stop exercising. There are lots of ways to stay motivated and engaged. Here are some examples. Enlist a family member or friend to exercise with you. Join or start a group or exercise class. Sign up for local exercise events. You can also get an app on your phone or computer to help you keep your goals and check-in. Some of these apps can be coordinated through health insurance plans and can lower health insurance costs. If you cannot afford local walks, runs or rides, then volunteer for one and often, you can get free entries to future events. It allows you to give back and set goals. Change up your exercise which will allow you to have more fun. Consider different activities during different seasons. Also, if you find yourself not engaged for a while, forgive yourself and start back up. It is ok to take a break, start over, and start something new.

Success is obtained through setting goals, developing an attainable plan, and persistence. You CAN do it! Live by example!

Live by example!

SECTION 3

EXERCISES TO CONSIDER

CHAPTER 7
EXERCISE BASICS

Recommended Time to Spend Exercising

The recommended time to spend exercising varies by age, goals of your exercise program and physical abilities. General recommendations for children and adolescents are for nearly double the activity of adults. Unless otherwise stated, the recommendations for exercise are general recommendations made from national organizations whose purpose is to study the benefits of exercise and active lifestyles on health. If you are over the age of 20 years old, your goal should be at least 30 minutes per day of exercise but try to incorporate at least moderate activity such as brisk walking on 3 of the days per week. The current recommendations by most medical organizations are that adults should get at least 150 minutes of moderate intensity exercise or 75 minutes of vigorous intensity exercise each week, preferably spread throughout the week. Moderate intensity can be as simple as walking a mile in approximately 20 minutes. Children and teenagers should get at least 1 hour of moderate intensity exercise daily with 3 of the days per week incorporating a more vigorous activity. The total time per day or per week can be split up into smaller increments which can have the same benefits over time. For instance 10 minutes of walking in the morning, 10 minutes at lunch and 10 minutes at the end of your day gets you 30 minutes total which is the minimum goal per day. Even if you do less than 10 minutes of exercise or activity in one setting, you can get substantial benefits over time. Some of the time spent doing exercises should includes performing strength training at least 2 non-consecutive days per week with 8-12 repetitions of each exercise and 8-10 different types of exercises that target all the major muscle groups. Older adults should do lighter weights or less resistance and increase the repetitions to 10-15 of each exercise still doing 8-10 different types of exercises that target all the major muscle groups. Sometimes getting started is the hardest step. Remember, even less than 10 minutes of exercise or activity can still provide significant benefits over time, so just get started.

Warm Up and Cool Down

Warming up prior to exercise is important for not only prevention of injuries during exercise but also for many of the health benefits received from exercise. Following exercise with a cool down period can further prevent injuries to the stress muscles endure during the more vigorous exercise session. To prevent injuries, always try to warm up your body for 2-3 minutes prior to starting an activity and cool down for 5-10 minutes after an activity. Examples of ways to warm up include slowly speeding up as you walk or cycle, swinging your arms back and forth, or marching in place. During the warm up, you are also increasing your heart rate to get to the target range you want to be at for your exercise. This is also when hormone production begins which can offer many of the benefits of exercising. Many of these hormones produced during your warm up are why you can get benefits from even less than 10 minutes of exercise. Ways you can cool down include slowing down your walk or cycling at the end of your session, stretching after your exercises, and slow deep breathing. The cool down session can be shortened if the total exercise session is less than 20 minutes.

Heart Rate Target During Exercise and for Fat Burning

It is important to get your heart rate to an optimum level for maximizing your exercise potential to achieve your overall goals as well as for staying in a safe target zone. A normal resting heart rate is between 60-100 beats per minute, bpm, although some people will have a heart rate slightly below 60 bpm. To calculate your maximum heart rate, subtract your age from 220. For instance, a 50 year old will have a maximum heart rate of 170 bpm. To calculate your target heart rate during exercise, multiple your maximum heart rate by 0.5 and by 0.85 which will give you the target range of 50-85% of your maximum heart rate. So a 50 year old will have a target heart rate range of 85-145 bpm during exercise which is 50-85% of their target heart rate. Fat burning typically happens at 60-70% target heart rate which you can calculate by multiplying your maximum heart rate by 0.6 and 0.7. Usually you will need to reach 60-70% of your target heart rate for at least 15 minutes to lose weight. So if weight loss is not a goal of yours, keeping your target heart rate at the lower target range, about 50%, will help prevent further weight loss. Make sure to review Chapter 5 if you are on medicines that may affect your heart rate as you calculate your goals.

Categories of Exercise

There are four exercise categories that are important which include the following: flexibility, balance, resistance or strength, and aerobic or endurance. Doing exercises in each of these categories will help stay overall fit, prevent injuries better, and benefit your overall health. Each category of exercises can promote different areas of health and wellbeing in different ways. For instance, flexibility exercises promote muscle and joint strength as well as flexibility. Aerobic exercise improves cardiovascular health. Both types of exercises can stimulate hormone productions at differing amounts to benefit other areas of wellness such as sleep, anxiety, depression, and pain.

I am going to give examples of different exercises in each of these categories that you could consider. This is not all inclusive. There are many other types of activities you could incorporate to fill in each category. Many times an exercise may involve multiple categories at once. For instance, yoga can involve flexibility, balance, resistance and endurance all at once depending on the type of yoga being done. Throughout further exercise descriptions, repetitions may be referred to as reps.

CHAPTER 8
FLEXIBILITY EXERCISES

Flexibility exercises help to strengthen muscles and joints and prevent injuries. Our flexibility helps us every day to do daily living activities as simple as getting a cup out of the cabinet, washing our hair, and putting on our clothes and shoes. Many different exercises can work on flexibility. Examples of some common flexibility activities include stretching, yoga, tai chi, and pilates. It is important to stretch all the different muscle groups to prevent injuries and improve exercise tolerance. For those under 65 years of age, it is recommended to hold a count of 30 seconds for each stretch, with a 10 second rest after the stretch before repeating the stretch. Try to repeat the stretch at least once initially (2 sets), working up to a goal of 4 sets. For those over 65 years of age, it is recommended to hold the stretch for 60 seconds for maximum benefit, with a 10 second rest after each stretch. It will usually take 6 weeks to start seeing the benefits of the flexibility exercises. Flexibility stretches are best done after you have warmed up a little with a short walk or marching in place for a couple of minutes. Also, while stretching, you should breathe regularly, not breath-hold. Shaking out the limbs between stretches can help keep the muscles warm and pliable.

If you are just beginning or have extra time, isolating the muscle groups may be easier. You can do individual stretches, where you focus on one muscle group at a time. If you have less time or are ready for a more challenging session, you can try to incorporate more complex stretching poses that will work multiple muscle groups at once. Exercises done in yoga and tai chi often move from one pose into another, essentially resting the muscle group during the transitions between poses. These activities will often include poses that work on strength and balance to provide more than one type of exercise at a time. Even if you have difficulty with standing or balance, you can often modify these exercises to be done while sitting in a chair.

These examples of flexibility stretches that follow are a good starting place to find a set of stretches for your exercise plan. When it says to hold the pose, then hold it for the appropriate time based on your age: 30 seconds if under 65 years old and 60 seconds if over 65 years old. When it says to repeat, then repeat the stretch up to 4 times, repeating with each side if the exercise focuses on left and right sides. Remember to breathe in and out regularly throughout these exercises, and avoiding breath-holding. Repetition is also called rep.

Flexibility Exercises that Isolate Muscle Groups

Neck Roll

Stand or sit with your back straight, arms down by your sides reaching towards the floor. Lean your left ear towards your left shoulder, relaxing the shoulders. Feel the stretch in your right neck. Hold the pose. Roll your head forward and towards your right shoulder with your right ear leaning towards the right shoulder. Hold the pose. Roll back to the left side to repeat the stretch.

Upper Shoulder Stretch

Stand or sit with your feet shoulder width apart. Raise your left arm straight out to shoulder height and reach your left arm across your chest towards the right shoulder, palm facing the floor. Reach up with your right arm to pull your left arm close to your chest, keeping your left arm straight. Hold the pose. Feel the stretch across the back of the left shoulder. Now switch arms and repeat. Hold the pose. Repeat the entire exercise. Picture below

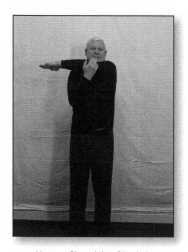

Upper Shoulder Stretch

Triceps Stretch

Stand or sit with your feet shoulder width apart. Raise your left arm straight up over your head, towards the sky. Then reach the left arm towards your right back; try to touch your right shoulder blade. You should feel the stretch in the back of your upper left arm. For extra stretch, you can pull your left elbow with your right hand towards your right shoulder. Hold the pose. Now switch arms and repeat. Hold the pose. Repeat the entire exercise. Picture below

To stretch both triceps at once, raise both hands straight up above the head and clasp your hands together. Relax your hands down towards your back shoulder blades and touch your thumbs to the middle of your back, pressing your elbows to the sky. Hold the pose.

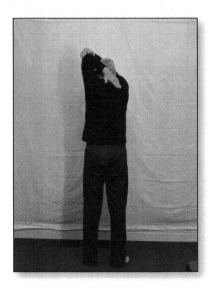

Triceps Stretch

Shoulder and Chest Stretch

Stand or sit with feet shoulder width apart. Clasp your hands behind your back and straighten your arms. Raise your hands as high as possible keeping your arms straight and hands clasped, bending forward at the waist if possible. (Do not bend if you are subject to dizziness or falls.) You will feel the stretch in your shoulders and chest. Hold the pose. Repeat. Picture below

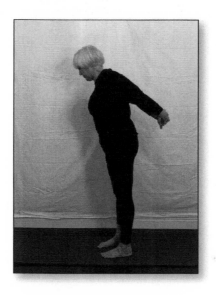

Shoulder and Chest Stretch

Low Back Stretch

Easy:

Stand or sit and reach both hands toward the sky, palms facing each other. Lean back slightly to feel a stretch in your low back. Look up to your hands as you lean back if you are not prone to dizziness. Hold the pose. Bring your arms down and place them on your knees if sitting or hang them straight down if standing and round out your back. Feel the stretch in your low back and along the sides of your back. Hold the pose. Repeat the entire exercise. Picture below

Hard:

Begin on your knees and place your hands shoulder width apart on the floor in front of you. Sit your buttocks towards your feet and feel the stretch in your low back and along the sides of your back. Hold the pose. Add to the stretch by moving your body weight up over your arms and round your back upwards pulling your stomach inwards to a pose that looks like a cat arching its back. Feel the stretch in your low back and along the sides. Hold the pose. Repeat the entire exercise.

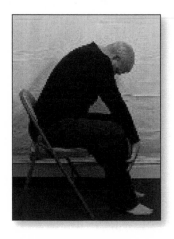

Low Back Stretch

Hip Flexor and Glute Stretch

Chair:

Sit in a chair with your feet hip distance apart in front of you.

If you can, lift your right foot and place it on your left knee and relax your right knee out so that the outside of your right ankle is resting on the top of your left knee, this will provide a good hip flexor stretch. Feel the stretch in your outer hip. Hold the pose. Repeat on the other side. Hold the pose. Repeat the whole exercise. Picture below

If you cannot lift your left foot, then sit forward at the front edge of a chair with your feet flat on the floor hip distance apart. Move your right foot back slightly to the outside of the chair. Your right foot toes will remain on the ground, but your right heel will come off the ground. Feel the stretch in your outer right hip. Hold the pose. Repeat on the opposite side. Hold the pose. Repeat the entire exercise. Picture below

Floor:

Sit on the floor with your legs straight out in front of you. Bend your left leg so that your foot is flat on the floor and place your left foot to the outside of the right knee. Turn and put your right elbow on the left knee so that your upper body is slightly twisted facing the left side of your body. Push your elbow against the outside of your left knee to get extra stretch in your hip and buttock. Keep your buttocks on the floor. Hold the pose. Repeat on the opposite side. Hold the pose. Repeat the entire exercise, each side.

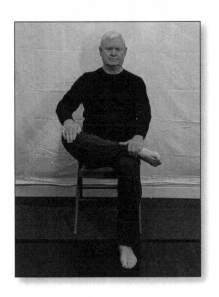

Hip Flexor and Glute Stretch

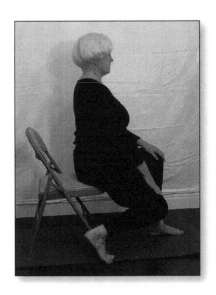

Adductor Leg Stretch

Stand with your feet wide apart. Hold on to a counter or chair for support if needed. Shift your weight to your right leg and slightly bend your right knee as you do this. Lean and reach towards your left leg, keeping your left leg straight and both feet flat on the ground the entire time. Feel the stretch in your inner upper thigh. Hold the pose. Repeat with the left leg. Hold the pose. Repeat the entire exercise, both sides. Picture below

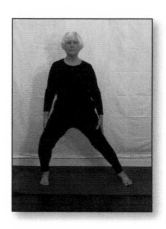

Adductor Leg Stretch

Hamstring Stretch

Standing:

Stand with your feet hip width apart facing a table or counter that is about hip height. Lean across the counter with your hands flat on the counter stretching out as far as you can. Slightly arch the lower back pressing your stomach towards the table. Feel the stretch in the upper back legs. For more stretch, pick a counter slightly below hip height or stand on a thick book or sturdy step to raise your hips slightly above the counter height. Hold the pose. Repeat.

Floor:

Lie on the floor on your back. Bend the left knee 90 degrees keeping the left foot on the floor. Raise the right leg straight up to the sky, keeping it as straight as possible. Keep your hips flat on the floor. Feel the stretch in the back of the raised right leg. Hold the pose. Repeat with the opposite leg. Hold the pose. Repeat the entire exercise. Picture below

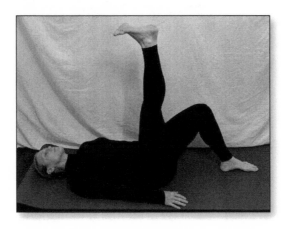

Hamstring Stretch

Quadriceps Stretch

Gentle Chair:

Stand up on the side of a chair and place your left knee on the chair holding on to the back of the chair with both hands. Gently lean back towards your buttocks to feel the stretch in your left quadriceps muscle. Hold the pose. Switch sides and repeat the exercise. Hold the pose.

Standing:

Stand up straight, feet hip distance apart. Hold a counter or chair for extra support. Bend your left leg back towards your buttock and grasp your left foot with your left hand. Stand up as straight as you can as you gently pull the left foot towards your buttock. Feel the stretch in the front of your upper left leg. Hold the pose. Repeat with the right leg. Hold the pose. Repeat the entire exercise. Picture below right

Floor:

Lie straight on your right side. Bring your left foot back towards your buttock and try to hold with your left hand. Feel the stretch in the front of your left upper thigh. Hold the pose. Repeat with the right leg. Hold the pose. Repeat the entire exercise.

Chair:

Sit up straight but move your buttocks so that your right buttock is slightly off the side of the chair. Reach down to grab your right foot with your right hand. Hold onto the chair with your left hand for support. Pull your right foot up towards your buttock until you feel a stretch in the upper part of your right thigh. You may not be able to get your foot off the floor for this. Hold the pose. Repeat with the left leg. Hold the pose. Repeat the entire exercise. Picture below

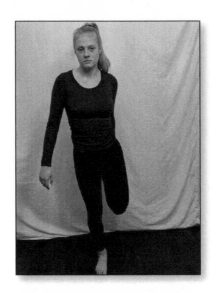

Quadriceps Stretch – standing

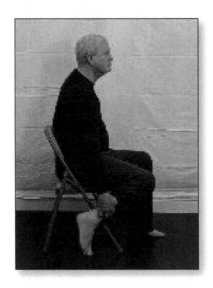

Quadriceps Stretch – gentle chair

Calf Stretch

Stand with both feet together and lean forward towards a wall or a counter until you feel a stretch on the lower back of your legs. Keep your feet flat against the floor. Hold the pose. Repeat.

You could do one foot at a time if it is easier for you.

Flexibility Exercises that Include Multiple Muscle Groups

Low Back/Hips/Hamstrings

Lie on your back on the floor with your feet straight out. Bring your left knee up to your chest and hug it into your chest. Hold the pose. Repeat with the right leg. Hold the pose. Repeat the entire exercise. Picture below

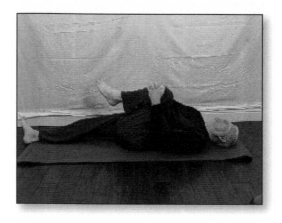

Low Back/Hips/Hamstrings

Low Back/Hips/Hamstrings/Glutes

Lie on back with feet flat on floor. Cross your left foot over or behind your right front thigh. Lift your right leg off of the floor and extend it straight into the air. Grab the back of your right leg and pull it towards your chest. Hold the pose. Repeat with the opposite side. Hold the pose. Repeat the entire exercise. Picture below

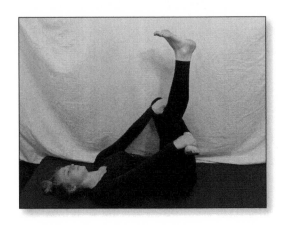

Low Back/Hips/Hamstrings/Glutes

Hip Flexors/Quadriceps/Back/Calf

Stand straight and take a big step forward with your right leg into a lunge bending your right knee. Keep the left leg straight behind you. Place your right hand on the floor, if you can, on the outside of your right knee and twist your upper body to the right as your reach your right arm to the sky. Hold the pose. Repeat on the opposite side. Hold the pose. Repeat the entire exercise. Picture below right

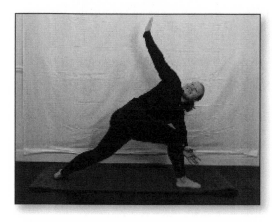

Hip Flexors/Quadriceps/Back/Calf

Low Back/Abdomen

Lie on the floor on your stomach with your legs straight. Raise your upper body onto your elbows which are shoulder width apart. Keep your palms flat on the floor in front of you so that your upper body rises off of the floor. Press your hips and thighs into the floor. For more of a stretch, straighten your arms to lift you higher off of the floor. Hold the pose. Repeat. Picture below

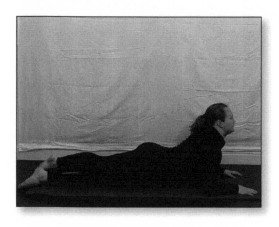

Low Back/Abdomen

Low Back/Hips/Obliques/Glutes/Quadriceps

Lie on your back with your legs extended straight onto the floor. Bring your left knee up to your chest. Hold pose. Then, relax the left knee to outside the right leg, extending the left leg straight for more of a stretch. Try to keep your back on the floor. For more of a spine stretch, turn your head to the left and stretch your arms out lateral in a T shape. Hold the pose. Repeat on the opposite side. Repeat the entire exercise. Picture below

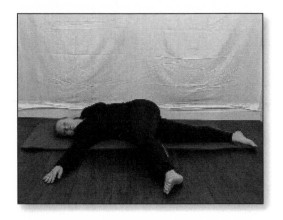

Low Back/Hips/Obliques/Glutes/Quadriceps

CHAPTER 9
BALANCE EXERCISES

Balance is important to prevent falls and injuries. We use balance in most of the activities of daily living that we do not even think about such as getting out of bed in the morning, preparing our meals, dressing, showering, and walking. As we bend, turn and move to do things, it requires balance. As we age, our balance is affected by many mechanisms, from medical problems to a lack of flexibility and strength. The activities that promote balance are as simple as walking on uneven ground or stairs, biking, standing on one leg at a time, skipping, and dancing. More structured activities such as yoga, tai chi and pilates can provide balance exercises that also help with flexibility and strength. Likely, the exercise routine you chose will allow you to easily incorporate motions that will improve your balance.

If you are prone to falls, try to incorporate more exercises that include balance as part of the exercise. In addition, try to do balance exercises every day. Some of the easiest to do on a daily basis is to walk up and down stairs but make sure you have a rail to hold on to if you are prone to falls. Also, standing on one leg at a time, raising the leg in the air higher, even potentially being able to hold it to your chest is another helpful exercise you can do for daily balance training. If you are limited to a chair, you can sit and do many yoga poses with your upper body that also help with balance.

Specific Balance Exercises

Look to the Sky

Stand up straight with your feet hip width apart. Look up towards the sky and hold that position for up to 60 seconds. Look straight ahead. Repeat.

Modification(s):
Raise your hands up over your head as you look up and clasp your hands together. When you look back straight bring your hand back down to your sides.

Keep your feet together instead of hip width apart.

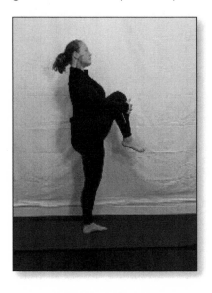

Standing on One Leg

Stand up straight with your feet together. Raise your right foot off of the floor and hold it for up to 60 seconds. Put it back on the floor and repeat on the other side. This completes 1 set.

Modification(s):

Lift your leg up until your quadriceps muscle is 90 degrees to the floor.

Lift your knee up to your chest and hug it. Picture above

Hold a chair to balance yourself if needed during the exercise.

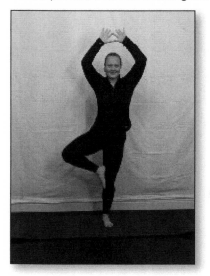

Standing on One Leg with Foot on Opposite Inner Leg

Standing on One Leg with Foot on Opposite Inner Leg

Stand up straight with your feet together. Raise your right foot off of the floor and place the bottom of your right foot onto the medial side of your left leg. Keep your hands palms together in front of your chest. Hold the pose for up to 60 seconds. Put it back on the floor and repeat on the other side. This completes 1 set.

Modification:

Raise your hands over your head with your hands clasped together. Look up at your hands if you can. Picture above

CHAPTER 10
RESISTANCE AND STRENGTHENING EXERCISES

There are a lot of ways to improve muscle mass which is necessary to protect the bones and joints of the body. Resistance and strengthening exercises can also stimulate hormone production which helps with wellness by improving sleep, lowering depressive and anxious feelings, and improving symptoms of pain. Keeping the muscles fit also helps with circulation and nerve function, lowers body fat, and improves cardiovascular fitness to help perform daily activities that require strength, like standing from a chair and lifting things. It is recommended by many health organizations to perform strength training at least 2 non-consecutive days per week with 8-12 repetitions of the specific exercise, incorporating 8-10 different exercises that target all the major muscle groups. Older adults should do lighter weights or less resistance and increase the repetitions to 10-15. This can be accomplished using body weight, resistance bands, free weights, medicine balls, or machine weights. By exercising the larger muscle groups first, the individual muscles are better warmed up for isolating single muscle exercises.

The major muscle groups include the chest, back, shoulders, biceps, triceps, abdomen, quadriceps and hamstrings. Various exercises can be done to focus on each of these muscle groups using body weight, resistance bands, machine weights, free weights, and medicine balls. Examples of the different exercises follow in this section. Many of the resistance band exercises described can be done without a band, or using a light free weight which can be hand weights or weights built into wraps that go around your wrist or ankle. When using machine or free weights, minimize each weight increase to less than 10% of the weight you are using. So for example, if you are using 20 pounds on a machine, an increase of 10% is adding 20 times 0.1 which is 2 additional pounds. This would be an increase from 20 to 22 pounds when you increase to the next amount you will use. Also, do not increase the weight until you can lift the current amount comfortably and for the desired repetitions for at least 2 training sessions. Perform strength training at least 2 non-consecutive days per week, performing 8-10 different exercises to cover all major muscle groups and plan to do 2-4 sets of repetitions. For those people who are younger, plan to do 8-12 repetitions and for those who are over 65 years old, plan to do 10-15 repetitions in each of the 2-4 sets. Typically doing 8-12 repetitions will allow you to build muscle faster than doing 10-15 repetitions. So if your goal is to stay lean and not necessarily build muscle, then do 10-15 repetitions keeping the weights a little lighter. Try to rest for at least 30 seconds in between exercise sets to allow your muscles to recover.

Repetition =rep

Specific Body Weight Resistance Exercises

Chest Exercises

Plank

Muscle groups: chest, shoulders, abdomen

Many exercises mentioned will start or use the plank or high plank position. This is an excellent core exercise if you hold the position for 30-60 seconds. Typically, this is where you start lying on your stomach flat on the floor. Place your hands palms flat on the floor next to your shoulders. Push your body up off the floor onto your elbows which are bent, palms flat on floor or hands made into a fist, with your body remaining flat, supporting your lower body on your toes. Hold the position for 30-60 seconds. Repeat for up to 4 reps. Picture below

Modification(s):
High plank is another common starting position for exercises. Instead of staying on your elbows, straighten your arms, locking your elbows into a high plank position. Picture below

Knee plank can be done with your arms on your elbows or straight in the high plank position. Stay on your knees as you push-up off the floor. The remainder of the exercise is done the same as the plank or high plank above.

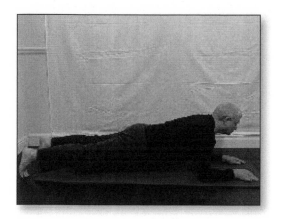

Plank

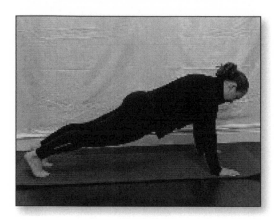

High Plank

Wall Plank

Stand with your feet hip-width apart facing a wall. Place your arms on the wall, shoulder-width apart and shoulder-height, straight out in front of you. Back your feet away from the wall so that you are leaning into the wall to provide some tension on your upper body and hold. Then walk your feet back forward so you can stand straight up to complete the rep.

Push-ups

Muscle groups: chest, back, shoulders, triceps

Using body weight, push-ups are a good way to focus on the chest, back, triceps, and abdomen muscles. A traditional push-up is done with your arms shoulder width apart, palms on the floor, abdomen tucked in and a flat back, legs off the floor and kept straight, then lowering your body weight with your arms bent until you are just above the floor in a plank-like fashion and then pushing up to straighten the arms. This is 1 rep. Try to keep your body as straight as possible throughout the push-up. Picture below

Modification(s):
Knee push-ups: Keep your knees on the floor as you push-up and lower your upper body. The remainder of the exercise is done the same as a standard push-up.

Alternatively, raise your buttocks to the sky slightly in a v shape, keeping your legs straight. The remainder of the exercise is done as a standard push-up. Start off the floor with your arms straight, then lowering your body weight bending your arms at the elbows until you approach but don't touch the floor, and then straighten your arms to complete 1 rep. Picture below

Stand up push-up: Stand away from the wall with your arms straight out, palms flat on the wall at shoulder height. Your feet should be shoulder width and positioned under your shoulders so that your trunk is straight. Then, lean towards the wall with your upper body keeping your back flat, bending your elbows until you approach the wall with your chest. Don't touch the wall with your body. Then push yourself back away, straightening your arms to complete 1 rep.

Challenge push-ups: Modify the standard push-up by widening your arms apart, or put them closer together to make a diamond with the fingers and thumbs of your 2 hands next to each other in the middle of your chest. Complete the motion of the push-up as you would with the standard push-up.

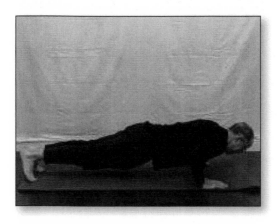

Push-up

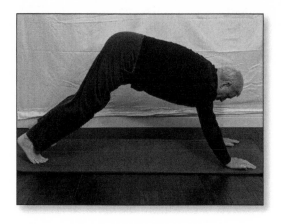

Modification of Push-up

Diamond Push-ups

Muscle groups: chest, back, shoulders, triceps

Start in a plank position off of the ground. Put your hands together on the floor with your first fingers and your thumbs together to make a diamond shape in line with the middle of your chest. Bend your elbows to lower your chest and torso to the floor, and then push back up straightening your elbows which is 1 rep. Picture below

Modification:
Keep your knees on the floor as you push up and lower your upper body. The remainder of the exercise is done the same as a diamond push-up. Start off the floor with your arms straight, then lowering your body weight bending your arms at the elbows until you approach but don't touch the floor, and then straighten your arms to complete 1 rep.

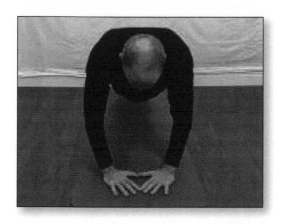

Diamond Push-up

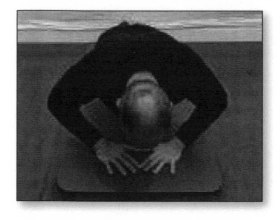

Diamond Push-up

Pull-ups

Muscle groups: chest, back

If you have access to a pull-up bar, then this is ideal for doing these exercises. A pull-up bar can be purchased that can fit over doorways inside the home. Often times they are available in parks. Also, keep in mind you may need to start on a stepping stool to assist yourself to do a complete pull-up. The goal is to have you hands on the bar just wider than shoulder width apart, starting with your arms straight as you hang from the bar and then pull yourself up until your chin touches or approaches the bar height.

Start the exercise by hanging from the bar, hands approximately shoulder-width apart, palms pointing away from you. As you pull yourself up towards the bar, exhale out a breath to tighten your abdomen and push your chest forward slightly, which will retract your shoulders back slightly, bending your elbows. Continue to pull up bringing your elbows in to your sides with the goal that your chin is slightly at the level of the bar. Slowly lower yourself to the hanging position inhaling a breath as you go down to complete 1 rep.

Modification(s):
Widen your hands, still with your palms facing away from you. Continue with the exercise as you would with the standard pull-up. Picture below

Center your hands next to each other, still with your palms facing away from you. Continue with the exercise as you would with the standard pull-up.

Use a chair to aid you in your pull-up if you cannot support all your own weight.

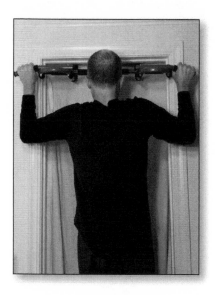

Pull-ups

Chin-ups

Muscle groups: chest, back, shoulders, biceps

Hang from the chin-up bar with hands shoulder width apart, palms facing towards you. Pull yourself up towards the bar, exhaling as you go, bending your elbows pulling them towards the sides of your body, reaching your chin towards the bar. Slowly lower your body back into the hanging position, inhaling as you lower yourself to complete 1 rep. Picture below

Modification(s):
Widen your hands, still with your palms facing towards you. Continue with the exercise as you would with the standard chin-up.

Center your hands next to each other, still with your palms facing towards you. Continue with the exercise as you would with the standard chin-up.

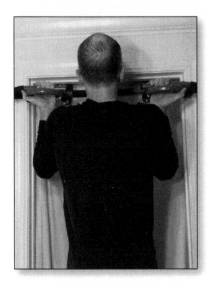

Chin-ups

Back Exercises

Swimmers

Muscle groups: back, abdomen, shoulders

Lie flat on the floor on your stomach with your arms straight over your head and legs straight. Raise your right arm and left leg off the floor. Hold at the top for up to 10 seconds with both limbs straight and then lower back down. Repeat with your left arm and right leg. That's one rep. Picture below

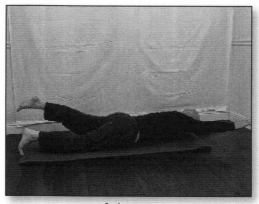

Swimmers

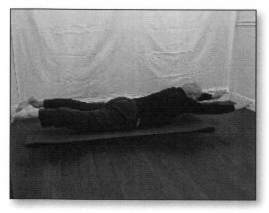

Flying

Flying

Muscle groups: back, abdomen

Lie flat on the floor on your stomach with your arms straight over your head and legs straight. Raise both arms and legs off the floor and hold for a count of 15-30 sec. Rest and repeat. Picture above

Shoulder Exercises

Arm Circles

Muscle group: shoulders

Arm circles are a good isolating shoulder exercise. Stand with your feet shoulder width apart, arms hanging at your sides. Raise your arms straight out like a scarecrow. Face your palms away from you with your fingers up and perform circles with both arms at the same time in the same direction, mimicking washing a window with your hand. Perform 20-30 circles. Reverse directions and perform another 20-30 circles. Start with small circles and then perform a separate set with larger circles to vary the exercise.

Pike Push-up

Muscle group: shoulders

Using body weight, pike push-ups are a good way to focus on the shoulders. This is a modification of a traditional push-up. Your arms are shoulder width apart, palms on the floor, abdomen tucked in. Move your feet and hands closer together to allow your buttocks to be high in the air with your body in a v shape. You lower your head towards your hands bending your elbows outwards, then push off the floor to straighten your arms to complete one rep. Your legs should remain straight as you do this exercise. Picture below

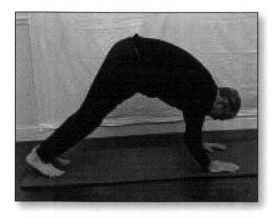

Pike Push-up

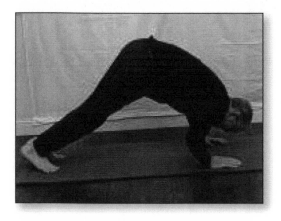

Pike Push-up

Bicep Exercises

Towel or Rope Bicep Curls

Muscle group: biceps, abdomen

Stand with your back straight against the wall, tightening your abs at the same time. Grab both ends of a long towel or rope with your palms facing upwards. Put one foot in the middle of the towel like it is a sling with your arms at your sides. It is best if your arms are able to remain straight when you put your foot into the sling. Make sure to keep your shoulders relaxed down and back against the wall. Bend your arms and pull your hands up against the resistance of your leg until your arm is at a 90-degree angle. Keep your upper arms stationary against the wall, with your elbows next to your body. Lower your leg back down to allow your arms to be straight to complete 1 rep. Picture below

Modification:
Perform the same exercise except when you pull your leg up to the 90-degree angle, hold this position against the resistance of your leg for a count of 30 seconds to complete 1 rep.

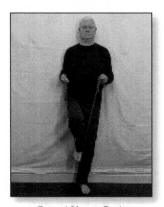

Towel Bicep Curls

Doorway Bicep Curls

Muscle groups: biceps, chest

Stand facing a narrow column with your legs shoulder-width apart. The wider your stance, the more difficult the exercise will be. Grab either side of the door frame with both hands at chest height. Your thumbs should be facing you pointed up and your arms should be nearly straight. Make sure to keep your shoulders relaxed down and back. Pull yourself forward until your chest nearly touches the door frame, and then push yourself back to the starting position straightening your arms to complete 1 rep. Picture below

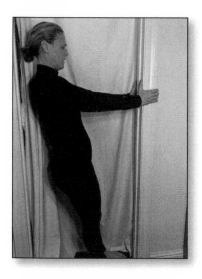

Doorway Bicep Curls

Triceps Exercises

Dips

Muscle group: triceps

Sit on a bench or in a sturdy chair with your legs bent or legs straight (harder) out in front of you. Starting with your elbows tight to your sides and your hands pointed forward, grip the end of the chair surface. Slowly lower your body down, bending your elbows straight back until they are bent about 90°. Lower for two seconds then push your body back up, locking out your elbows at the top, and repeat. Make sure to keep your body close to the chair and do not go too deep, or this can cause injury to your shoulder.

Modification(s):
Straighten your legs and complete the remainder of the exercise the same way. Picture below

Straighten your legs and lift one up straight in the air and alternate legs every 3-5 reps. Complete the remainder of the exercise the same way. This will also exercise your abs.

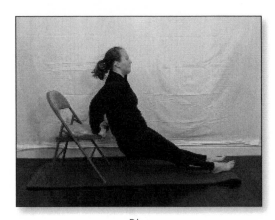

Dips

Crab Walk

Muscle group: triceps, abdomen, hamstrings

Sit on the floor with your legs bent in front of you, feet flat on the floor and shoulder width apart. Place your hands with palms flat on the floor just behind your hips. Push up with your hands to straighten your arms and raise your abdomen into the air, flattening your abdomen as much as possible. Adjust your wrists slightly to make sure it is comfortable. Walk your hands and feet backwards like a crab for 20-30 paces. Repeat up to 4 times. Picture below

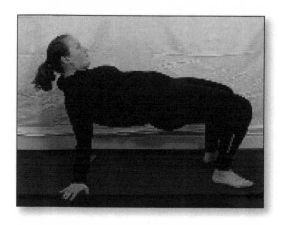

Crab Walk

Plank to Push-up

Muscle groups: triceps, abdomen

Start in a plank position on your elbows instead of with your arms straight. Have your hands in front of you palms down in a 90-degree angle. Drive your forearms into the ground and push your body up straightening your arms to get onto the palms of your hands. Hold the position for up to 10 seconds and then drop back down to your forearms, keeping your body flat and off of the ground to complete 1 rep.

Modification:
Stand facing a wall, feet shoulder width apart, far enough away from the wall that your arms are straight and your palms are able to be flat on the wall, shoulder width apart. Lean towards the wall until your elbows are touching the wall then slowly push yourself back away from the wall to complete 1 rep.

Press up

Muscle groups: triceps, abdomen

Lie flat on the ground on your stomach with your hands, palms down, next to your shoulders. Push-up with your hands straightening your arms, raising your upper body without completely locking your elbows to allow tension on your triceps. Slowly return to the starting position to complete 1 rep.

Abdomen Exercises

Crunches

Muscle group: abdomen

Start lying on your back with your legs bent at about 90-degree angle and your feet flat on the floor. Clasp your hands behind your head with your elbows out to the sides. Slowly raise your upper chest towards the ceiling until your back comes off of the floor. Then lie back to the floor to complete 1 rep. Picture below

Modification:
Challenge yourself more by touching your right elbow to your left knee and then your left elbow to your right knee and continue to alternate as you come up for each crunch. Picture below

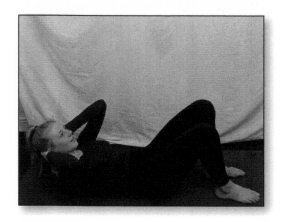

Crunches

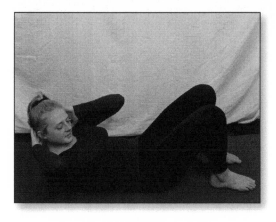

Crunches

Reverse Crunches

Muscle group: abdomen

Start lying on your back with your legs together straight out on the ground. Raise your legs up into the air, keeping your back and buttocks on the ground and feet flexed. You can simply hold this position for a count of 30-60 seconds or you can slowly lower your legs back to just above the ground to complete 1 rep, raising them again in the air to repeat the exercise. Picture below

Modification:
When your flexed feet are in the air, hold the position and crunch your abdomen to allow your buttocks to rise off the floor slightly and push your feet further towards the sky. These are small crunches but are challenging. Picture below

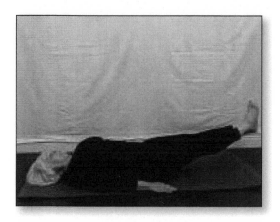

Reverse Crunches

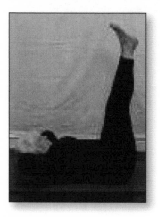

Reverse Crunches – Modification

Standing Sit-ups

Muscle group: abdomen

Stand with your feet hip-width apart, hands clasped behind your head with your elbows pointing out to the sides. Lift your left knee bending at the waist to touch it to your right elbow, and then put your leg down. Do the opposite side, lifting your right knee to touch it to your left elbow and put your leg back down to complete 1 rep. Picture below

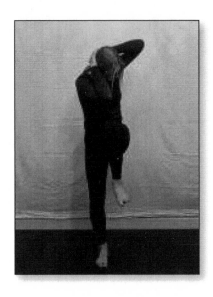

Standing Sit-ups

Standing Oblique Crunches

Muscle group: abdomen

Stand with your feet hip-width apart, hands clasped behind your head with your elbows pointing out to the sides. Lift your right knee bending at the waist to the side reach towards your right elbow, and then put your leg down. Do the opposite side, lifting your left knee towards your left elbow and put your leg back down to complete 1 rep. Picture below

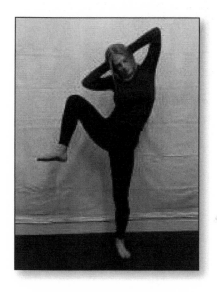

Standing Oblique Crunches

High Plank

Muscle groups: chest, shoulders, abdomen

Many exercises mentioned will start or use the plank position. This is an excellent core exercise if you hold the position for 30-60 seconds. Typically, this is where you start lying on your stomach flat on the floor. Place your hands palms flat on the floor next to your shoulders. Push your body up off the floor, straightening your arms, locking your elbows with your body remaining flat, supporting your lower body on your toes. Hold the position for 30-60 seconds. Repeat for up to 4 reps. Pictured previously

Modification(s):
Stay on your knees as you push-up off the floor. The remainder of the exercise is done the same.

Rest your body in the same position on your elbows in a 90-degree angle with your palms flat on the floor.

Plank Shoulder Taps

Muscle group: abdomen

Start in a high plank position on your hands. Tap each hand to the opposite shoulder engaging your abdomen to keep your hips as still as possible. Tapping both shoulders is 1 rep. Picture below

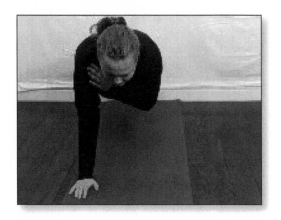

Plank Shoulder Taps

Side Plank Body Rotations

Muscle group: abdomen

Start in high plank position on your hands. Rotate your entire body to the right side onto your right arm stacking your feet, and lift your left arm up into the air towards the ceiling into a side plank. Keep your body straight throughout the exercise. Rotate back to the standard plank position and then rotate your entire body to the opposite, left side, onto your left arm, lifting your right arm up into the air towards the ceiling into a side plank. That is 1 rep. Picture below

Modification:
As you are in the side plank position, raise your leg into the air instead of stacking your feet.

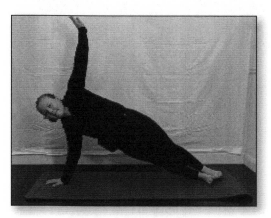

Side Plank Body Rotations

Side Plank Dips

Muscle group: abdomen

Start in a side plank position either high plank or on your elbow as described above with your feet stacked. Drop your hip towards the floor, not touching the floor, and then raise it back into the starting position or a little higher if you can. That is 1 rep. Repeat on the opposite side. Picture below

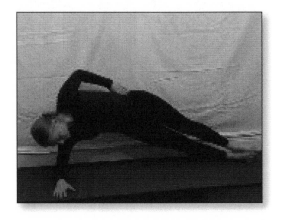

Side Plank Dips

Twists (also known as bicycle)

Muscle group: abdomen

Sit on the floor with your knees bent. Lift your feet into the air and mimic bicycling with your legs. Your hands should rest behind you on the floor. Each rotation of both legs is 1 rep.

Modification(s):
Lift your hands straight into the air as you bicycle your legs.
Put your hands behind your head with your elbows out and twist your torso as you bicycle your legs to meet your elbow with the opposite leg, right elbow touching left knee, then left elbow touching right knee. Picture below

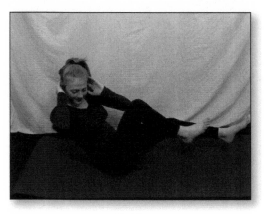

Twists

Alternating Knee-to-Chest Twist

Muscle group: abdomen

Sit with your legs straight out in front of you. Lift your legs off the ground and bring one of your knees up to your chest, holding it with your arms and try to touch the knee with your nose. Then switch legs. Keep your legs off the ground as you extend the leg back outwards after you hug it to your chest. You can alternatively do this in a lying position with you back flat against the floor as you perform the same motions with your legs. One rep is after you have brought each leg to your chest. Picture below

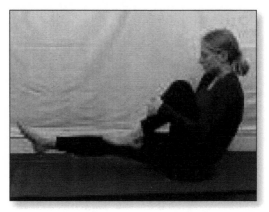

Alternating Knee-to-Chest Twist

Single or Double Leg Lifts

Muscle group: abdomen

Lie flat on your back with your legs straight out, hands next to your hips with your palms on the floor. Lift both legs off the floor slightly. Keep your low back pressed into the floor. Raise 1 leg up into the air keeping it as straight as possible with your foot flexed, and then bring it back down to the starting position as you raise the opposite leg up. Scissor them back and forth. Lifting and lowering both legs is considered 1 rep.

Modification:
You can also bring both legs up together, keeping them straight and feet flexed then slowly bring them back to just above the floor before repeating the exercise. Picture below

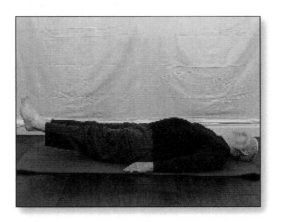

Double Leg Lifts

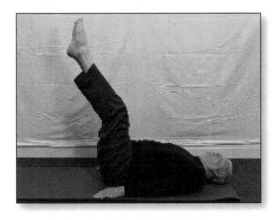

Double Leg Lifts

Quadriceps Muscles

Wall Sits

Muscle groups: quadriceps, hamstrings

Stand with your back flat against a wall with your feet hip width apart. Walk your feet forward as you bend your knees until you are in a sitting position, knees at an approximate 90 degrees angle, with your back still flat against the wall. Try not to hold the wall with your hands. Hold the position for up to 1 minute. Repeat up to 4 times. Picture below

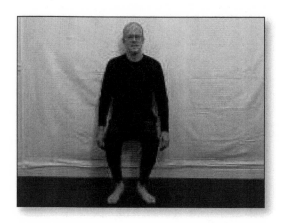

Wall Sits

Squats

Muscle groups: quadriceps, hamstrings

Start standing with your feet shoulder width apart. Drop your bottom towards the ground until your knees are both bent about 90-degrees and your fingertips can touch the floor. Then push off the heels to stand up and complete 1 rep. Rise up onto your toes when you stand up out of the squat for an added exercise for your calves. Picture below

Modification:
Chair squats: Start sitting in a chair. Stand up without pushing off of the chair if possible. Then sit down to complete 1 rep. You can challenge yourself more by doing this with 1 leg at a time.

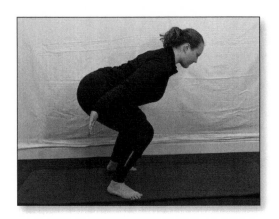

Squats

Squat Jumps

Muscle groups: quadriceps, hamstrings, abdomen

Start standing with your feet shoulder width apart. Drop your bottom towards the ground until your knees are both bent about 90-degrees and your fingertips can touch the floor. Then push off with both feet to jump into the air, reaching your hands to the sky. Come back down with your feet shoulder width apart to repeat the exercise again.

Single Leg Squats

Muscle group: quadriceps, hamstrings, abdomen

Start standing with your feet shoulder width apart. Put your right leg straight out in front of you just off the floor. Bend your left leg 90-degree angle into a squat, keeping your arms out in front of you for balance. Push off the heel of your left leg to come back into a standing position which completes 1 rep for that leg. Switch legs in between reps, or after you have completed all the reps for that leg. Picture below

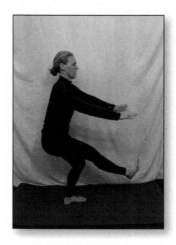

Single Leg Squats

Squatting Lunges

Muscle groups: quadriceps, hamstrings

Start standing up with your legs wide apart. Drop your bottom towards the floor, bending your knees and lightly touching the floor with your fingertips. Walk your hands towards your right foot until your left leg is straight. Then walk your hands towards your left foot until your right leg is straight. That is 1 rep. To make it more challenging, lift your straight leg slightly off the floor before you move back towards the opposite leg. Picture below

Modification:
Start in the squatting lunge position holding the back of a chair before you drop your bottom into the squatting position. Use the chair to balance yourself as you move from side to side straightening your leg.

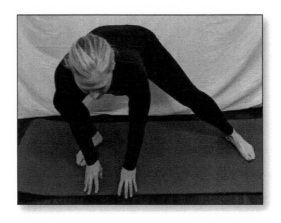

Lunges

Lunges

Muscle groups: quadriceps, hamstrings

Stand with your feet together and your arms hanging at your sides. Step straight forward with your right foot until your right knee is at a 90-degree angle with the floor. Your back left knee should not touch the floor. Then, push off with your right front leg to bring your back left leg back to a standing position. Repeat with the opposite left leg to complete 1 rep. Picture below

Modification:
Stand holding the back of a chair. Step back with your left leg until the right knee near the chair is bent into a 90-degree angle. Step your left leg towards the chair until you are in a standing position and repeat with the opposite right leg.

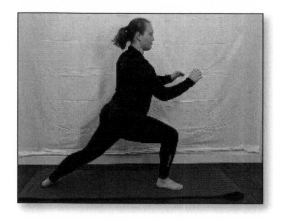

Squatting Lunges

Side Lunges

Muscle groups: quadriceps, hamstrings

Start in the same position as the standard lunge. Instead of stepping straight forward, step forward at about a 45-degree angle to
the side, bending your knee until it is at a 90-degree angle with the
floor. Then push back with your bent knee leg to bring your legs back
together at the same spot you started at to complete 1 rep with that
leg. Alternate your left and right legs.

Reverse Lunges

Muscle groups: quadriceps, hamstrings

Start by standing with your feet hip width apart. Step backwards with
your left foot bending both knees which will be 90-degrees. Return
to standing by pushing through your right heel to bring your left leg
forward. Repeat on the other side to complete 1 rep.

Hamstring Muscles

Hip Raises

Muscle groups: hamstrings, abdomen, back

Lie on your back with your knees bent, hip-width apart, feet flat on the ground. Keep your arms straight at your sides next to your body. Push down through your heels to raise your hips off the floor, flattening your torso. Slowly lower your hips towards the floor to complete 1 rep. Picture below

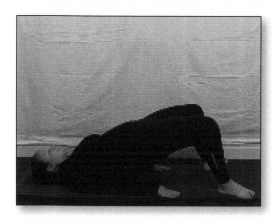

Hip Raises

Single Leg Hip Raises

Muscle groups: hamstrings, abdomen, back

Start like you did for the standard hip raises. Lift your right leg straight up above you with the toes pointing to the ceiling. Raise your hips and then lower them back down keeping your leg in the air. That is 1 rep for that leg. You could do all the reps for each leg before switching to the other side or alternate legs in between each rep. Picture below

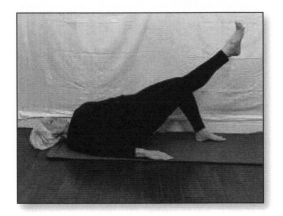

Single Leg Hip Raises

Back Kicks

Muscle group: hamstrings

Start on the ground on all fours, on your knees which should be hip-width apart and hands which should be shoulder width apart. Pull your left knee towards your chest, keeping your foot flexed. Then kick your left leg back behind you and toward the sky, then back down to the ground. Switch and do the other leg to complete 1 rep. Picture below

Modification:
Start standing up with your legs together, and then bend forward at the waist with your hands slightly forward for balance. Kick your leg backwards into the air with the foot flexed to complete 1 rep for that leg. You can hold onto a chair for balance.

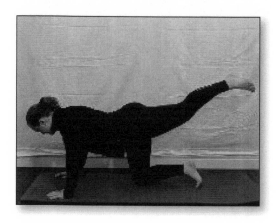

Back Kicks

Resistance Band Exercises

The exercises discussed here will be described using a band, but you can do many of these exercises with free weights, or without weights, or without a band at all. You may even want to start without a band or weight until you feel strong enough to add them. There are many different bands you can get to do these exercises. There are bands that have handles and those that are just strips of flexible material. The material can be in a tube formation or flat. The bands also come in different tension to mimic using weights for strengthening. You do not need a lot of tension to get benefit with these exercises. Pick a set of bands that you prefer. Be careful with the ones with handles since sometimes the handles can break, especially when they get older although having a handle to hold on to can make it easier to use. You can get the bands at sporting goods stores and large department stores. When anchoring your band, either loop it around a solid structure or tie it tightly around the structure. Examples of solid structures include a column in your house or a pole or post outside. You can also have someone hold the end of the band for you which is what we did for these pictures.

If you decide to use no bands or you decide to use weights, mimic with your arms and legs the motion you would do if you had a band when doing the exercise. Free weights can be hand weights that you hold or you can get weights that are built into wrist bands or ankle bands that wrap around your wrists and ankles, respectively. You do not need a lot of weight with most of these exercises so a 1 to 3 pound added weight can be plenty. Always start with a lower weight and slowly add more in a controlled manner.

Chest Exercises

Standing Chest Press

Muscle group: chest

Anchor the band around a sturdy column at chest height. Face away from the column. Stand with your feet shoulder width apart with a staggered foot stance, with your left foot slightly in front of you. Grab both ends of the band (or if you have tied off the band, then the single end) with your right hand, palm facing down. Bring your arm up into a bent position slightly below shoulder height. You can keep your left arm straight down next to you or point your left arm straight out in front of you. Move your right arm in a punching motion forward, to meet your left arm if it is also raised, and then slowly allow it to return to the bent position. That is 1 rep for that arm. Complete all your reps in that set before switching arms. Picture below

Modification:
This can be done seated in a chair. You must anchor the band at shoulder height for when you are seated.

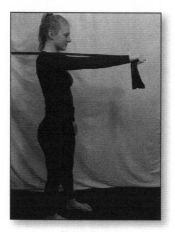

Chest Press

Chest Press at an Incline

Muscle group: chest

This exercise is just like the chest press with a band except you are pointing at the sky at an approximate 45-degree angle. Anchor the band around a sturdy column at chest level. Face away from the column. Stand with your feet shoulder width apart with a staggered foot stance, with your left foot slightly in front of you. Grab both ends of the band (or if you have tied off the band, then the single end) with your right hand, palm facing down. Keep your left arm at your side or bring your left arm up to a 45 degree angle pointing at the sky. Move your right arm in a punching motion forward, meeting your left arm at a 45 degree angle if it is also raised, and then slowly allow it to return to the bent position. That is 1 rep for that arm. Complete all your reps in that set before switching arms. Picture below

Modification:
This can be done seated in a chair. You must anchor the band at chest height for when you are seated.

Press the band towards your arm at the same angle, and then slowly allow it to return to the bent position. That is 1 rep for that arm. Complete all your reps in that set before switching arms.

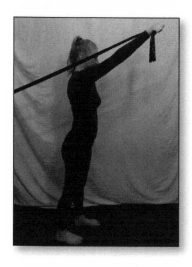

Chest Press at an Incline

Chest Press at a Decline

Muscle group: chest

This exercise is just like the chest press with a band except you are pointing at the floor at an approximate 45-degree angle. Anchor the band around a sturdy column at eye-level height. Face away from the column. Stand with your feet shoulder width apart with a staggered foot stance, with your left foot slightly in front of you. Grab both ends of the band (or if you have tied off the band, then the single end) with your right hand, palm facing down. Either keep your left arm at your side or point your left arm down to a 45 degree angle pointing to the ground. Move your right arm in a punching motion forward, meeting your left arm at a 45 degree angle if it is raised, and then slowly allow it to return to the bent position. That is 1 rep for that arm. Complete all your reps in that set before switching arms. Picture below

Modification:

This can be done seated in a chair. You must anchor the band at eye level when you are seated.

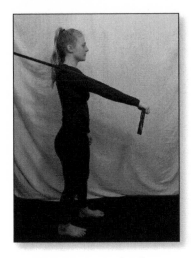

Chest Press at a Decline

Chest Fly

Muscle groups: back, chest

Variation 1:

Secure the band at medium height in front of you. Stand with feet shoulder-width apart and slightly staggered, one foot in front of the other. You can be slightly bent over keeping your back straight. Hold one end of the band in each hand, palms facing each other, arms extended straight out in front of you. Pull the band back with both arms to the sides of your body, bending your elbows 90-degrees, pressing your shoulder blades together, and keeping your back straight throughout. Hold for 2-3 seconds before returning your arms to their starting position to complete 1 rep. Picture below

Modification (s):

Chair: Sit at the edge of a chair with your legs together, knees bent 90-degrees in front of you. Loop the band under your feet and grab an end with each hand, palms facing together. Lean forward over your knees slightly keeping your back straight. Keeping your arms slightly bent at the elbows, pull the bands back to the sides of the body bringing your shoulder blades together. Hold for 2-3 seconds before returning your arms to their starting position to complete 1 rep.

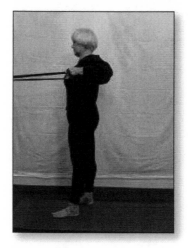

Chest Fly – Variation 1

Chest Fly – Variation 2:

Muscle group: chest

Secure the band at chest height on your left side. Stand with your legs shoulder width apart. Grab the band with your right hand, palm facing down, with your right arm extended across your chest starting from the left side of your body. Keeping your elbow straight, pull the band horizontally across your chest extending your arm fully out to the right side of the body. Your left hand is resting on your hip throughout the motion. Slowly allow it to return to the starting position to complete 1 rep. Complete all your reps in that set before switching arms. Picture below

Modification:

This can be done seated in a chair. You must anchor the band at chest height for when you are seated.

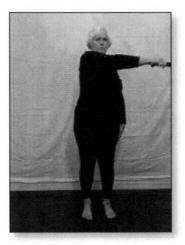

Chest Fly – Variation 2 (start)

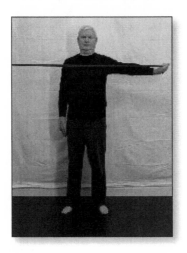

Chest Fly – Variation 2 (end)

Chest Fly at an Incline

Muscle group: chest, back, triceps

Secure the band at thigh height on your left side. Stand with your legs shoulder width apart. Grab the band with your right hand near your left hip, palm facing down standing up straight. Your left hand is resting on your left hip. Pull upwards on the band at a 45 degree angle until it is in front of your chest keeping your right arm as straight as possible. Slowly allow it to return to the starting position to complete 1 rep. Complete all your reps in that set before switching arms. Picture below

Modification:
This can be done seated in a chair. You must anchor the band at low height for when you are seated.

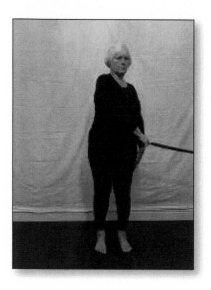

Chest Fly at an Incline (start)

Chest Fly at a Decline

Muscle group: chest, back, triceps

Secure the band at a high height on your right side. Stand with your legs shoulder width apart. Grab the band with your left hand, extending your left arm out to the right side at shoulder height, palm facing down. Your right hand is resting on your hip. Pull the band until it is in front of your abdomen keeping your left arm as straight as possible. Slowly allow it to return to the starting position to complete 1 rep. Complete all your reps in that set before switching arms. Picture below

Modification:
This can be done seated in a chair. You must anchor the band at high height for when you are seated.

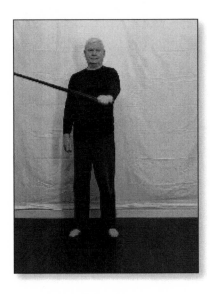

Chest Fly at a Decline (end)

Pull-over

Muscle group: chest, shoulders

Anchor the band at a low position. Face away from the anchor and lie on your back. Grab the free end of the band with both hands, stretching your arms straight out behind your head just above the floor. With your elbows slightly bent, pull the band overhead until it is above your chest, reaching towards your knees until you meet resistance. Slowly return the band to the starting position to complete 1 rep. Complete all your reps in that set before switching arms. Picture below

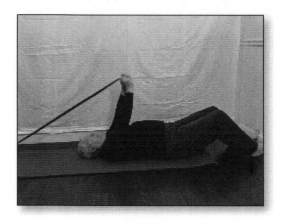

Pull-over

Back Exercises

Pull-a-parts

Muscle group: back

Stand or sit with your feet shoulder-width apart. In each hand, hold one end of the band so that it is stretched across the front of your body. Palms should be facing inwards and elbows should be straight throughout the exercise. Stretch your arms straight out in front of you at shoulder-height. Squeeze your shoulder blades together as you stretch your arms out to the sides of your body, still at shoulder height. Hold for 2-3 seconds then relax back to the starting position to complete 1 rep. Picture below

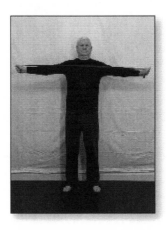

Pull-a-parts

Seated Row

Muscle group: back

Sit on the edge of a chair with your legs straight or partly bent in front of you. Put the band around the bottom of your feet, holding one end of the band in each hand. Sit up straight. Squeeze your shoulder blades together and pull your elbows straight back as far as possible with a goal of your hands next to your chest. Hold the position for 2-3 seconds then relax back to the starting position to complete 1 rep. Picture below

Modification:
Sit on the ground with your feet straight out in front of you, bands looped under your feet, one band in each hand. Sit up straight. Complete the exercise as above.

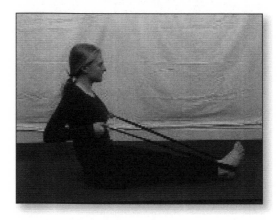

Seated Row

Standing Row

Muscle group: back

Secure the band low in front of you as you stand with your feet shoulder width apart, slightly staggered one in front of the other. Hold one end of the band in each hand, palms facing each other and arms extended straight in front of your hips. Pull the bands back towards your abdomen and hold for 2-3 seconds before relaxing back to the starting position to complete 1 rep.

Modification(s):
Do one arm at a time, resting your other arm on the opposite leg or hip during the exercise.

You can also position your body in a partial lunge with the band looped under your front foot. Have one end of the band in each hand and complete the exercise as above. Picture below

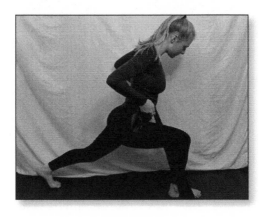

Standing Row

High Row – Seated

Muscle group: back

Secure the band high. Sit in a chair with your legs in front of you bent at 90-degrees. Grab an end of the band with each hand in front of your head with your arms extended, palms facing each other. Pull the handles back slowly towards your abdomen, holding the pose for 2-3 seconds. Then allow them to slowly return to complete 1 rep. Picture below

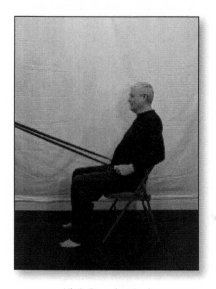

High Row Seated

Pull-down

Muscle group: back

Anchor the band up high overhead. Pull the free ends down next to your sides as you kneel facing the anchor so the bands are in front of you. Grip each end of the band with your arms extended overhead and hands slightly wider than shoulder-width, palms facing each other. Keep your elbows slightly bent and pull the band down toward the floor while contracting your back muscles. Once your hands reach your shoulders, slowly raise then back to the starting position to complete 1 rep. Picture below

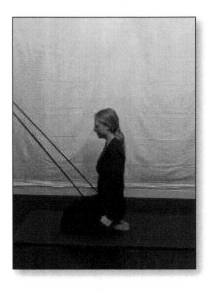

Pull-down

Shoulder Exercises

Overhead Press

Muscle groups: shoulders, back

Stand with your feet shoulder-width apart with the band under your feet. Grasp each end of the band with each hand positioning your hands at shoulder level with palms facing each other and elbows against your chest. Press straight up with your arms rotating your palms forward as you fully extend your arms. Hold for 2-3 seconds before slowly returning to the starting position to complete 1 rep. Picture below

Modification:
You can do this from a seated position either sitting on the band or preferably, placing the band under your feet and leaning forward just slightly to be able to press straight upwards. The remainder of the exercise should be followed as outlined above.

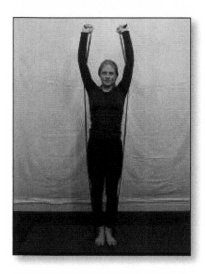

Overhead Press

Forward Shoulder Press

Muscle groups: shoulders, back

Stand with your feet staggered, one in front of the other. Secure the band under your back foot and grab each end with a hand resting over your shoulders with your elbows bent and palms facing forward. Push the bands up and forward until your arms are fully extended. Pause there briefly before you allow them to slowly return to just above your shoulders to complete 1 rep. Picture below

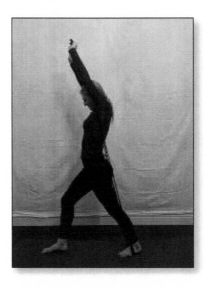

Forward Shoulder Press

Forward Raise

Muscle group: shoulders

Stand with your feet shoulder-width apart, with the band under your feet. Grasp the end of the band with your right hand, palms facing in or down. Bring your right arm straight out in front of you to shoulder height without locking the elbow, but keeping the arm straight. Slowly lower the right arm back down to complete 1 rep. Complete all the reps in that set on the right arm before switching to the left. Picture below

Modification:
This can be done in a chair. Sit at the edge of a chair and loop the band under your feet. Continue the remainder of the exercise as outlined above.

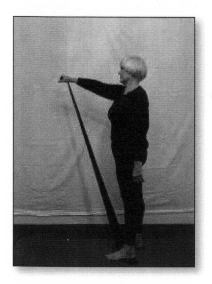

Forward Raise

Lateral Raise

Muscle group: shoulders

Stand with your feet shoulder-width apart, band under your feet. Grip each end of the band with each hand, arms down by your sides and palms facing in. Raise your arms straight out to shoulder –level and hold it for 2-3 seconds. Elbows can be bent slightly. Slowly lower back down to the starting position to complete 1 rep. Picture below

Modification:

This can be done in a chair. Sit at the edge of a chair and loop the band under your feet. Continue the remainder of the exercise as outlined above.

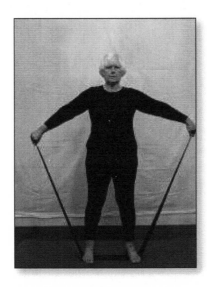

Lateral Raise

Upright Row

Muscle group: shoulders

Stand up straight with feet shoulder-width apart, positioned over the center of the band. Grip each end of the band with your hands, palms facing your body just in front of your thighs. Pull the band straight up in front of your body to the shoulder level, keeping your elbows bent and positioned in a 'v' shape. Slowly lower the band back to the starting position to complete 1 rep. Picture below

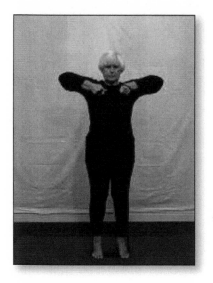

Upright Row

Internal Band Shoulder Rotation

Muscle group: shoulders

Secure your band at medium height on your left side. Stand with your left hip towards the band with your feet shoulder width apart. Grab the handle (or both ends) with your left hand, arm bent at the elbow 90-degrees with your hand in front of your abdomen, palm facing towards you. Keep your upper arm pressed against your side and your elbow bent. Pull the handle in towards your abdomen, pause briefly. Then allow the band to slowly return to the starting position to complete 1 rep. Complete all the reps in a set on one side before switching to the opposite side. Keep your elbow bent and arm pressed against your abdomen throughout the exercise. Picture below

Modification:

This can be done while you are sitting in a chair.

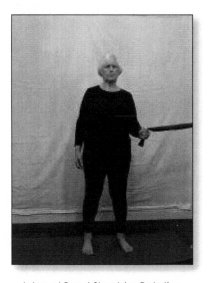

Internal Band Shoulder Rotation

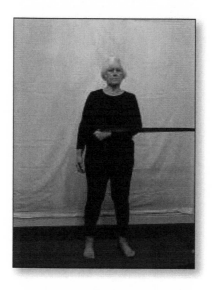

Internal Band Shoulder Rotation

External Band Shoulder Rotation

Muscle group: shoulders

Secure your band at medium height on your left side. Stand with your left hip towards the band with your feet shoulder width apart. Grab the handle (or both ends) with your right hand, forearm resting across your abdomen, elbow bent 90-degrees, palm facing towards you. Rotate your right arm out away from your body until it is pointing straight away from you, keeping your upper arm pressed against your side and your elbow bent. Then allow the band to slowly return to the starting position to complete 1 rep. Complete all the reps in a set on one side before switching. Picture below

Modification:
This can be done while sitting in a chair with your knees bent 90-degrees in front of you.

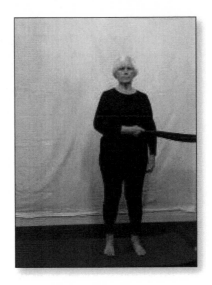

External Band Shoulder Rotation

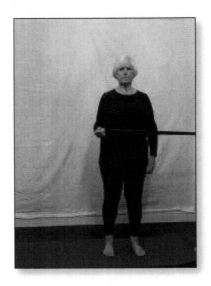

External Band Shoulder Rotation

Bicep Exercises

Standing Biceps Curl

Muscle group: biceps

Stand with your feet shoulder width apart with both feet placed over the middle of a band. Grab a handle in each hand, starting with your arms down at your sides. With your palms facing away from you, keeping your upper arms next to your sides, curl your arms upwards towards your shoulders, bending your elbows. Pause briefly before you extend your arms back to the starting position to complete 1 rep. Picture below

Modification:
This can be done while sitting in a chair. Keep your back straight while performing the reps.

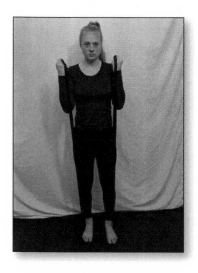

Standing Biceps Curl

Concentration Curls

Muscle group: biceps

Start in a forward lunge with your body, left leg in front with the band under your left foot. Grab one end of the band with your left hand, resting your left elbow on the inside of your left knee. With your palm facing away from your knee, curl the band upwards toward your left shoulder and squeeze your bicep at the top of the curl, just before you are about to touch your shoulder. Then slowly lower your arm back down to the starting position to complete 1 rep. Complete all the reps in a set on one side before switching arms. Picture below

Modification:
This can be done in a chair. With your feet shoulder width apart, secure the band under your right foot. Lean forward until your right elbow rests just on the inside of your right knee. Grab one end of the band with your right hand and complete the exercise as outlined above.

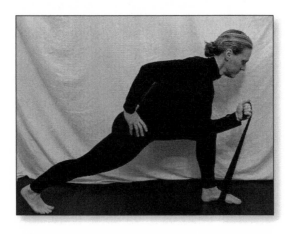

Concentration Curls

Wrist Curl

Muscle group: forearm

Sit in a chair with your feet shoulder width apart. Secure the band under your left foot. Rest your right elbow on your right thigh near your knee and hold the band with your right hand, palm facing up. Keep your forearm still during this exercise, Curl your hand up at the wrist, pausing briefly at the top of the curl. Then slowly return your wrist and hand to the starting position to complete 1 rep. Complete all the reps in a set on one side before switching wrists. Picture below

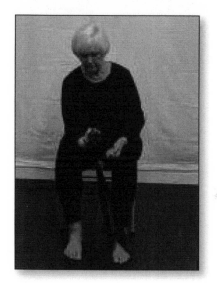

Wrist Curl

Wrist Extension

Muscle group: forearm

Sit in a chair with your feet shoulder width apart. Secure the band under your right foot. Rest your elbow on your left thigh near your knee and hold the band with your left hand, palm facing down. Pull the band upwards by extending your wrist upwards, pausing briefly at the top of the curl. Then slowly return your wrist and hand to the starting position to complete 1 rep. Keep your forearm still throughout this exercise. Complete all the reps in a set on one side before switching wrists. Picture below

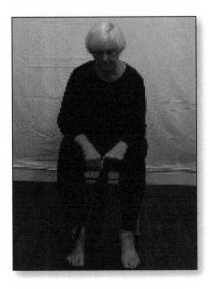

Wrist Extension

Triceps Exercises

Triceps Kickback

Muscle group: triceps

Stand in a forward lunge with your right foot in front, looping the band under your right foot. Hold each end of the band, positioning your upper arms at your sides, elbows bent 90-degrees, with your palms facing behind you. Straighten your arms, extending your forearms backwards, palms facing the sky. Pause briefly before returning your arms back to the starting point to complete 1 rep. Alternate legs between sets. Picture below

Modification:
Sit in a chair with your legs shoulder width apart, feet in front of you. Secure a band under your right foot. Lean forward, resting your left arm across your thighs and grab the band with your right hand. Keeping your upper arm against your side, palm facing behind you, straighten to extend your arm behind you. Pause briefly before returning to the starting position to complete 1 rep. Complete all the reps in a set on one side before switching sides.

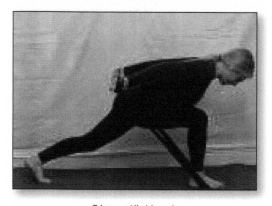

Triceps Kickback

Overhead Triceps Extension

Muscle group: triceps

Standing with your feet slightly staggered, band looped under your back foot; grab each end of the band with a hand, arms next to your sides. Extend your arms up straight over your head with your palms facing forward. Slowly allow the band to pull your hands backwards, palms facing the sky as you bend your elbows 90-degrees. Then, slowly extend the arms straight again over your head to complete 1 rep. Try to keep your elbows pointing forward, not to the sides, during the exercise. Picture above right

Modification:
Sit in a chair with the band under your glutes. Complete the exercise as outlined above.

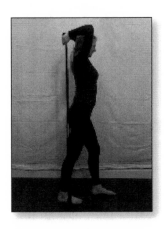

Overhead Triceps Extension

Abdomen (Abs) Exercises

Kneeling or Standing Crunch

Muscle group: abs

Attach the band to a high anchor, like the top of a door. Grasp both ends of the band in your hands, kneeling or standing to face the bands and bring them to the center of your chest, allowing your elbows to flare out to the sides. Hold the bands securely and crunch forward towards your hips, contracting your abs. Slowly return to the starting position to complete 1 rep. Picture below

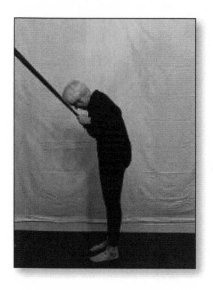

Standing Crunch

Woodchoppers

Muscle groups: abs, back, legs

Attach the band to a high anchor. Stand with your right side to the anchor, feet shoulder width apart. Grab the free ends of the bands with your arms stretched over your head, and bring your hands together. In a continuous motion, pull the band down and across your body to the front of your left knee, rotating your hips and pivoting your left foot. Bend your knees as your reach to the left knee to add more resistance and leg exercise. Slowly allow the band to retract back up to the starting point to complete 1 rep. Switch sides after you complete all the reps on that side. Picture below

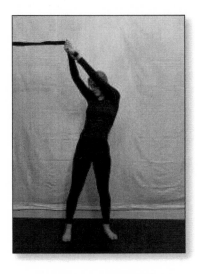

Woodchoppers – step 1

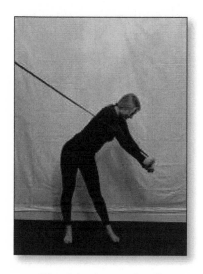

Woodchoppers – step 2

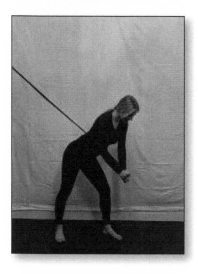

Woodchoppers – step 3

Squat Sideways Walking

Muscle groups: abs, legs

Anchor a band on a column or support slightly below your chest level. Grasp the ends until there is tension on the band. Squat like you are sitting in a chair. Hold the bands with both hands straight out in front of your chest and step laterally until the band is too tense to go any further. Slow and controlled, side step back to center and then go the other direction and back to center to complete 1 rep on each side. Keep your core tight and remain in a squat throughout the exercise. Picture below

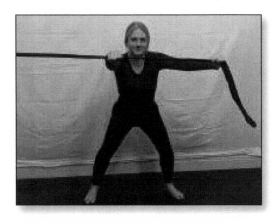

Squat Sideways Walking

Reverse Crunch

Muscle group: abs

Anchor the band on a low support. Lie on your back with your knees bent 90 degrees and wrap the band around your feet. Move away from the support until there is tension on the band. Keep your back flat against the floor and pull your knees toward your shoulders, contracting your abdominal muscles. Slowly return to the starting position to complete 1 rep. Picture below

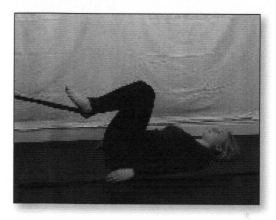

Reverse Crunch

Twists

Muscle group: abs

Sit on the floor with your legs extended wrapping the center of the band around the bottom of your feet. Hold the free ends of the band with both hands. Slightly bend your knees, keeping your feet on the floor, and lean back about 45 degrees. Rotate the band to your right hip, bringing your left hand across your body. Then rotate towards your left hip bringing the right arm across your body. Bring your arms back to center to complete 1 rep.

Modifications:

You can raise your legs slightly off the floor during the exercise for an added challenge. Picture below

You can substitute a weight for the band.

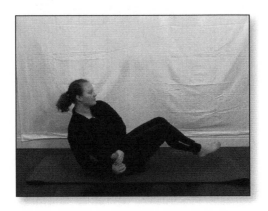

Twists

Trunk Rotations

Muscle groups: abs, back

Secure the band at a medium height. Stand with your legs shoulder width apart and grab the band with both hands, arms extended out in front of your chest. There should be some tension on the band. Rotate your upper body to the left and then slowly return to your start position before rotating your upper body to the right. Slowly return to the start position to complete 1 rep. Picture below

Modification:

Sit in a chair at the edge of the seat with your feet hip width apart on the floor in front of you and then perform the exercise the same as above.

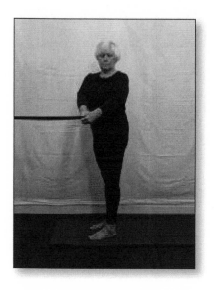

Trunk Rotations

Low to High Trunk Rotations

Muscle groups: abs, back

Secure the band low. Stand with your legs shoulder width apart and grab the band with both hands, arms extended out in front of your hips. While rotating your body to the left, bring your arms up to your left keeping them extended. Hold the position for a few seconds, and then slowly return to the starting position before repeating the same exercise in the opposite direction which will complete 1 rep. Picture below

Modification:

Sit in a chair at the edge of the seat with your feet in front of you on the floor in front of you and then perform the exercise the same as above.

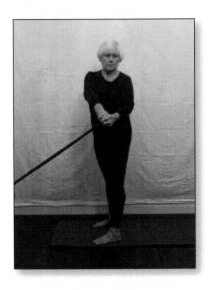

Low to High Trunk Rotations

Side Bend

Muscle group: lateral abs

Secure the band up high. Stand sideways with your right side towards the band, feet shoulder width apart. Grab the band with both hands, arms extended above your head. Tilt your upper body to the left, away from the band, and slowly bring it back to the starting position to complete 1 rep. Complete all the reps of that set before switching sides. Keep your arms extended throughout the exercise. Picture below

Modification:

Sit in a chair instead of standing. Perform the exercise the same otherwise.

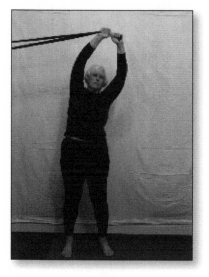

Side Bend

Quadriceps Exercises

Front Squat

Muscle groups: quadriceps, hamstrings, glutes, abs

Stand on the band with your feet slightly more than shoulder width apart. Hold a band in each hand and bring the top of the band over the back of each shoulder. You could alternatively hold a band in each hand and cross your arms across your chest. Squat down like you are going to sit down, chest up, abs firm with a goal of squatting to a 90 degree angle with the floor. Hold the position briefly before rising back up to the starting position to complete 1 rep. Picture below

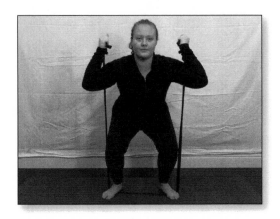

Front Squat

Leg Extension

Muscle group: quadriceps

Anchor a loop of your band in a low position and loop the other end around your left ankle, facing away from the band. Step away from the anchor to create tension on the band. Position your feet hip-width apart and shift your weight to the right foot. Lift the left leg off the floor and extend the knee and leg until it straightens out in front of you. Hold the position briefly before returning slowly to the start position to complete 1 rep. Complete all reps on 1 side before switching sides. Hold a wall next to you for balance if needed. Picture below

Modification:

Sit in a chair towards the edge of the seat. Secure 1 loop of the band under a foot of the chair or on a low position behind the chair. Loop the other end of the band around your ankle. With your leg hip width apart in front of you, starting with your feet flat on the floor, extend the leg with the loop around your ankle in front of you, engaging the quadriceps. Hold the position briefly before returning to the starting point to complete 1 rep. As above, complete all reps in the set before your switch sides.

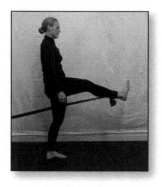

Leg Extension

Prone Leg Curl

Muscle groups: quadriceps and hamstrings

Anchor the end of the band to a door or support. Lie on your stomach, belly down with the band around your right ankle. Scoot away from the anchor to create tension. Tighten your core and bend your right leg at the knee, bringing your heel toward your glutes as far as you can. Slowly return your leg to the starting position to complete 1 rep. Complete all the reps on 1 side before switching sides. Picture below

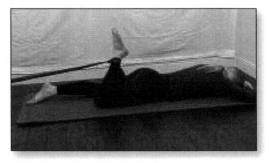

Prone Leg Curl

Bridge

Muscle groups: quadriceps and glutes

Tie a band to your legs right above your knees. Lie on your back with your feet on the floor bending your knees to 90 degrees. Rise up with your hips until your body is flat, contracting your glutes throughout the exercise. Hold the position for a few seconds before slowly relaxing back to the starting position to complete 1 rep. Picture below

Modification:

Pull your knees apart while you are in the bridge position for an added challenge.

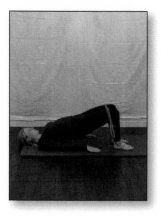

Bridge

Standing Abduction

Muscle group: quadriceps

Anchor a band at ankle height to a support and loop it around your left ankle. Stand with your right side facing the support and step away to create some tension. Start with your feet together. Then lift your left foot slightly off the floor and laterally extend your leg away from the support. Slowly return the leg to the starting position to complete 1 rep. Complete all the reps on 1 side before switching sides. Hold on to a wall or chair for support if needed. Picture below

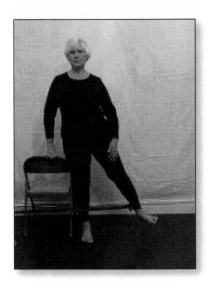

Standing Abduction

Seated Abduction

Muscle group: quadriceps

Sit at the edge of a chair and tie a loop band around both legs, just above the knees. Place your feet slightly wider than your shoulders. Slowly press your knees out, turning your feet in as your legs move apart. Hold for a few seconds before returning your knees back together to complete 1 rep.

Standing Adduction

Muscle group: quadriceps

Anchor a band at ankle height to a support and loop it around your left ankle. Stand with your left side facing the support and step away to create some tension. Start with your feet together and then step away from the support with your right foot to create a wider stance. Use a chair or wall if needed to add support. Then lift your left foot slightly off the floor, shifting your weight to the right leg. Bring your left leg to meet your right leg and then return to the starting point to complete 1 rep. Complete all the reps on 1 side before switching sides. Picture below

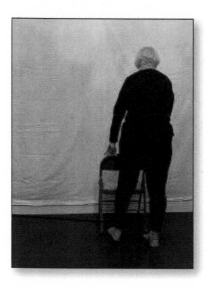

Standing Adduction

Lateral Walk

Muscle groups: quadriceps, glutes

Tie a band around your lower legs, just above your ankles. Start with your feet shoulder-width apart in a half squat. There should be tension on the band the entire time. Step with short steps sideways to the left 8-10 steps and then to the right 8-10 steps to complete 1 set. Picture below

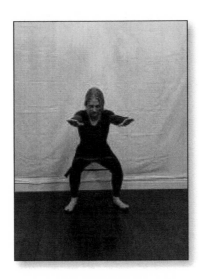

Lateral Walk

Lunges with a Band

Muscle groups: quadriceps, hamstrings, glutes

Secure the band underneath your right foot that is forward in front of you. Step back with your left foot, the opposite foot, into a lunge position. Your right knee should be at a 90 degree angle to the floor. Hold an end of the band in each hand and bring your hands up to your shoulders with your palms facing forward. Push yourself up by extending your legs and then return to the lunge position to complete 1 rep. Keep your foot with the band under it in the same place throughout the reps. Complete all the reps in 1 set with the left leg forward before switching to the right leg. Picture below

Modification:
When you are in the lunge position, push-up with the bands extending your arms into the sky and then slowly return your hands back to the shoulders to exercise your back, triceps and core.

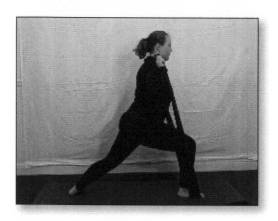

Lunge with a Band

Hamstrings and Lower Leg Exercises

Ankle Eversion

Muscle group: hamstrings and calf muscles

Sit on the ground with your feet extended in front of you. Keep your feet next to each other and wrap a band around your feet near the toes. Pull the toe area of your feet away from each other by stretching the band and then slowly return your feet together to complete 1 rep. Keep your heels pressed together throughout the exercise.

Calf Raises

Muscle groups: calf and shin muscles

Sit in a chair and loop a band around the toes of your foot. Pull upwards on the band to provide tension on the band. Lift your toes of the foot upward keeping your heel on the ground and then press the toes back to the floor to complete 1 rep. Complete all the reps on 1 foot before switching.

Modification:

Sitting on the floor with your feet extended in front of you, loop the band around one the toes of one foot. Pull tension on the band while your toes are flexing towards your upper body. Now extend your foot like you are pressing a pedal, and then slowly bring the foot back to the flexed position to complete 1 rep. Complete all the reps on 1 side before switching feet.

Machine-based Exercises

Follow the guide on the machine you are using or work with a trainer at the gym you attend to be sure you are using the machine appropriately. Each machine is slightly different. I will list examples of exercises for each major muscle group to consider for a complete body work out.

Chest Exercises

Seated Chest Press

Bench Press

Back Exercises

Rowing Machine

Lateral Pulldowns

Shoulder Exercises

Rowing Machine

Shoulder Press

Bicep Exercises

Cable Curls

Triceps Exercises

Press downs

Abdomen Exercises

Seated Abs Machine

Quadriceps Exercises

Leg Extension

Leg Press

Hamstring Exercises

Leg Curls

Free weights

Free weights can be very beneficial but do require some instruction to make sure the exercise is done appropriately so that you do not overstress your muscles. Many free weight exercises should be done with someone else who can spot you as you lift the weights to help if you cannot complete the exercise. I will list some examples of types of exercises, but I would encourage you to have a trainer at a gym teach you the appropriate techniques and be available to spot you while doing free weights.

Chest Exercises
Bench Press

Back Exercises
Fly
Upright Rows
Bent Over Rows

Shoulder Exercises
Dumbbell Lateral Raise
Shoulder Shrugs

Bicep Exercises
Curls

Triceps Exercises
Kickbacks

Abdomen Exercises
Weighted crunches

Quadriceps Exercises
Squats (with weights)
Lunges (with weights)

Hamstring Exercises
Stiff-leg Deadlifts

CHAPTER 11
AEROBIC AND ENDURANCE

Aerobic and endurance exercise has many health benefits. It is important for cardiovascular and pulmonary health. Also, during aerobic or endurance exercising, your body produces hormones that help with wellness such as improving sleep, decreasing anxiety and depression, improving pain and preventing and fighting cancer. The current recommendations by most healthcare organizations are that adults should get at least 150 minutes of moderate intensity exercise or 75 minutes of vigorous intensity exercise each week, preferably spread throughout the week. If you are over the age of 20 years old, your goal should be at least 30 minutes per day of exercise, incorporating at least moderate activity such as brisk walking on 3 of the days per week. The total time per day or per week can be split up into smaller increments. For instance 10 minutes of walking in the morning, 10 minutes at lunch and 10 minutes at the end of your day gets you 30 minutes total which is the minimum goal per day. But it has been shown that even exercising less than 10 minutes can benefit you. So if you are just getting started, or having limitations from your cancer diagnosis or treatment, it is important to do some amount of aerobic type activity.

To prevent injuries, always try to warm up your body for 2-3 minutes prior to starting an activity and cool down for 5-10 minutes after an activity. Examples of ways to warm up include slowly speeding up as you walk or cycle, swinging your arms back and forth, or marching in place. Ways you can cool down include slowing down your walk or cycling at the end of your session, performing some stretching after your exercise session, and slow deep breathing.

It is important to get your heart rate to an optimum level for maximizing your exercise potential. A normal resting heart rate is between 60-100 beats per minute, bpm, although some people will have a heart rate slightly below 60 bpm. I will review how to calculate your maximum, target and fat burning heart rate goals. To calculate your maximum heart rate, subtract your age from 220. For instance, a 50 year old will have a maximum heart rate of 170 bpm. To calculate your target heart rate during exercise, multiple your maximum heart rate by 0.5 and by 0.85 which will give you the target range of 50-85% of your maximum heart rate. So a 50 year old will have a target heart rate range of 85-145 bpm during exercise which is 50-85% of their maximum heart rate (170 bpm). Fat burning typically happens at 60-70% maximum heart rate which you can calculate by multiplying your maximum heart rate by 0.6 and 0.7. Usually you will need to reach 60-70% of your target heart rate for at least 15 minutes to lose weight.

There are many different exercises that can get your heartrate up for developing endurance. The easiest, and probably cheapest, is simply walking. Other popular types of exercises include jogging, running, biking, and swimming. Sometimes, these activities are unable to be done easily outside for various reasons, such as weather or location. Also equipment limitations will affect what exercise you do. Many of these exercises will offer benefits that help in other exercise categories, such as walking on uneven surfaces can help with balance, as can biking. Swimming is great for strengthening the upper and lower body. I will provide some examples of other activities that can be partnered together to get your heart rate up to your goal without leaving your house.

Aerobic Exercises

Jumping Jacks

Stand with your arms by your sides and legs together. Jump in the air slightly as your widen your legs apart, slightly wider than shoulder-width and at the same time clap your hands together over your head. Then, jump again as you bring your legs back together and hands back to your sides to complete 1 rep.

Squat Jacks

Start with your feet together and your hands at your chest. As you jump your feet apart slightly wider than shoulder-width, squat slightly at the same time as if you were going to sit in a chair and raise your arms out to the sides. Then jump your feet back together and return to a standing position to complete 1 rep.

Plank Jacks

Start in a high plank position: body straight, hands on the floor, palms flat, body slightly raised above the floor with your abs tightened to keep your back flat. Keeping your abs tightened, jump your feet out a little wider than shoulder-width apart and then back together to complete 1 rep.

Mountain Climbers

Start in a high plank as described previously under plank jacks. Draw your right knee under your chest. Then straighten it out and return it to the floor behind you as you bring your left knee into your chest. Keep switching your legs as if you are running in place although you can modify the speed. Picture below

Modification: Standing in place with your legs hip-width apart, raise your left arm above your head towards the sky as you raise your right leg up, knee towards your chest. Then bring your leg and arm down and raise the opposite right arm and left leg up similarly as if you were climbing up the side of a mountain.

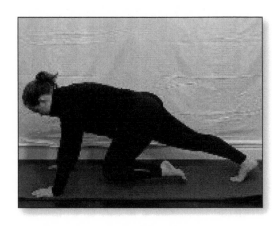

Mountain Climbers

Burpees

Stand with your feet shoulder-width apart, arms by your sides. Bend your knees as you reach forward to place your hands on the floor in front of you. Kick your legs straight out behind you and then start lowering your body to the ground, bending at the elbows into a push-up. Push your body back up quickly away from the floor and hop back up into a standing position jumping into the air, reaching your arms up into the sky. End with your knees slightly bent to complete 1 rep. Picture below

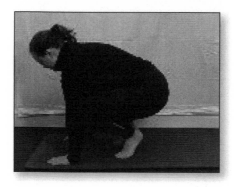

Burpees – position 1

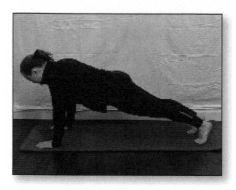

Burpees – position 2

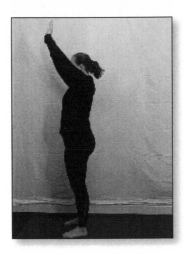

Burpees – position 3

Marching in place

Start standing up with your legs together and arms at your side. Then, lift your right knee towards your chest and at the same time raise your left arm towards your left shoulder. Then lower your right knee and left arm. Now raise your left leg towards your chest and at the same time raise your right arm towards your right shoulder before lowering it and repeating back to the opposite side.

Butt Kicks

Stand with your feet hip-width apart and start jogging in place. Allow your feet to come up behind you high enough to tap your butt, if you can.

Frog Jumps

Start in a partial squat position. Swing your arms behind your hips. Then push off your heels and jump forward, land on both feet, and then immediately sink back into a squat position and jump again. Picture below

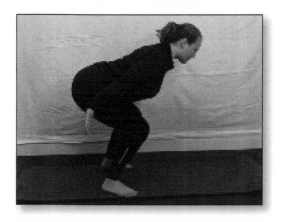

Frog Jumps

Jump Rope

Use a long rope or heavier weighted band if you do not have an actual jump rope. Even if you do not have a rope, you can mimic holding a jump rope and still get the same exercise. Jump rope faster to increase your heart rate more.

Bunny Hops

Stand with your feet together and hop in place, or back and forth over a line. You can do big hops or smaller hops.

SECTION 4

SPECIFIC AREAS OF INTEREST

CHAPTER 12
BREAST CANCER

Exercise can improve recovery from breast cancer treatments, improve the tolerability of the treatments and lower the risk of developing a new or recurrent breast cancer. As previously outlined in this book, exercise improves health and wellbeing in numerous ways which can lower the risk of cancer, including breast cancer, and can help both recover from and tolerate the treatments for breast cancer such as surgery, radiation, chemotherapy and hormonal therapy. Whether you have had breast cancer and are recovering from or going through treatments, or whether you want to avoid breast cancer altogether, exercise should be an important part of your daily routine.

Breast cancer treatments can affect people in many ways depending on the treatments received. Some people only require surgery, but others require radiation, chemotherapy and/or hormonal therapies. And then there are people who are focused on preventing breast cancer altogether. This chapter will go into more detail on how exercise can specifically prevent breast cancer, and how it benefits those recovering from treatments for breast cancer, going through treatments for breast cancer, or living with breast cancer. For those who have received treatments for breast cancer, there are considerations when exercising that will be outlined in this chapter. At the end of the chapter, I will outline an example work out plan for someone recovering from breast cancer treatments.

After what you have read so far in this book, if you are still wondering
how exercise can prevent breast cancer, then let's cover some of
the specifics again. There are higher rates of breast cancer associated with obesity, and exercise decreases obesity rates. There is also
a slightly higher rate of breast cancer in women with diabetes, and
exercise has been shown to lower the rates of diabetes and control
blood sugar better in those who have diabetes. Studies have proven
that those who exercise regularly have lower rates of breast cancer
occurrences and recurrences. Yes, regular exercise lowers the rates
of breast cancer.

When looking at the types of exercise that are beneficial, nearly all
types have shown to lower the rates of breast cancer including aerobic exercise such as walking, and also exercises such as resistance
training and yoga or stretching. One might wonder how stretching
can prevent breast cancer, but when you think about the hormonal
effects of actively using your body as we discussed in Section 1 of this
book, it can start to make sense. Insulin-like growth factor very likely
plays an important role and is lowered with any type of activity, even
stretching, which may inhibit cancer cell development. Other hormones including testosterone, growth hormone, thyroid hormone,
epinephrine and insulin are involved with strengthening muscles and
joints, managing the body's metabolism, and maintaining appropriate weight. Together, the hormones produced during exercise promote wellness of the body and likely all contribute to the lower rates
of breast cancer.

Other hormones that are produced during exercise called endorphins are also increased in the blood of people who participate in
vigorous exercise. Remember that these hormones are structurally
similar to morphine and can activate opioid receptors in the brain

and elsewhere to minimize pain which may be how they improve arthritis pain and scar tissue pain. In addition, exercise can improve and prevent pain by strengthening the muscles that support the joints putting less stress on those joints. Risks of fractures are reduced by having stronger muscles and healthier joints. Recall also that exercise helps improve coordination and flexibility of the body which can lower the risk of falls. Better body mechanics promote health, lowering injuries, and improvement and prevention of pain.

Keeping these health benefits in consideration when planning the types of exercises to incorporate into your routine will help you come up with a successful program which should include aerobic exercises, resistance or strength training, and stretching. Balance exercises can be incorporated into some of the activities to simplify your routine. The aerobic exercises should be aimed at attaining and maintaining a normal weight.

For those who have undergone treatment for breast cancer, there are certain muscle group exercises that are important to improve recovery and long-term wellbeing. Surgery can leave lasting physical changes including scar tissue which can cause tightness of the skin and joints, often referred to as contractures, and swelling of the arm and chest called lymphedema. Radiation can also lead to similar physical changes. Usually, it is recommended to not do any significant exercises of the upper body until you have healed adequately from surgery, at least 4-6 weeks. And then, once you start upper body exercises, start slow and proceed as your body is ready so that you do not cause the surgical incision site to heal more slowly. In addition, radiation may slow your ability to progress with your exercises during the treatments, but you can still incorporate a stretching program during the radiation. The radiation can cause tightness of the skin and local tissues, and it can take 6 to 12 months, even sometimes longer, for that tightness to resolve. Stretching your upper body which includes your arm, shoulder, back and chest will be important in your exercise routine and should be done at least 4-5 days per week, and I would suggest daily. Find a time to set aside to do them as part of your daily routine so that you do not forget, such as when you take your shower or just prior to going to bed. Also, remember to use sun screen when you are in the sun for up to 12 months after radiation as your skin is more sensitive to the sun. Wearing adequate undergarments when you exercise so that you have good upper body support is important during exercise.

If you are exercising while receiving chemotherapy, then it is important to know the side effects of the specific medicines you are receiving when considering your exercise routine. If the chemotherapy you are receiving can cause fatigue, weakness, or dizziness which all can occur with anemia, then shorten your aerobic exercise that you do at any given time to shorter more frequent intervals at slower paces and make sure to hydrate well prior to, during and after you exercise. In this situation, you may also need to do less weight or resistance when doing strengthening exercises. You can still stay toned by doing more repetitions of lighter weights during this time. If the chemotherapy you are receiving lowers your immune system, then be careful working out with crowds, like at gyms or in large groups. Chemotherapy often leads to bowel changes such as constipation or diarrhea, and sometimes nausea and even vomiting. Staying well hydrated will help with these side effects. Often exercise will actually make these side effects better. There are some types of chemotherapy given for breast cancer that can cause numbness and tingling in the hands or feet. Being careful with balance exercises during this time is important, but exercise can actually often improve these symptoms as well.

Most chemotherapy will make you more sensitive to the sun for at least 6 months and up to a year, so wear sunscreen when you are in the sun for more than about 10 to 15 minutes depending on your skin type. Fair complexions may require sunscreen for even a few minutes of sun exposure. Chemotherapy can cause dry skin and sometimes rashes; excessive sweating can worsen those conditions. Make sure to moisturize your skin. You may need to do short intervals of aerobic exercise to minimize sweating until you have recovered from these side effects of chemotherapy.

Hormonal therapy treatments if indicated to treat your breast cancer can sometimes make menopausal symptoms worse and sometimes cause weaker bones while you receive them. It may surprise you, but exercise has also been shown to improve menopausal symptoms such as hot flashes, irritability, depression, anxiety, and arthritis pain associated with menopause. This is felt to be from the increased healthy and safe hormone production produced during exercising that we discussed above, as well as increased serotonin and norepinephrine during exercise which improve depression and anxiety, improve sleep and offer a sense of wellbeing. Often regular daily aerobic exercise alone can manage menopausal symptoms without the need of additional supplements or medicines. Incorporating some strengthening, flexibility and balance exercises will help keep the bones strong and prevent falls and fractures. Often weight gain can be seen while on hormonal therapy treatments or in the first 1 to 2 years after completion of chemotherapy which can be countered by regular aerobic exercise focusing on keeping your target heart rate range in the 60% to 70% of your maximum heart rate range for at least 15 minutes per session where fat burning occurs.

So what might an exercise plan look like for someone who has received treatment for a breast cancer which included surgery followed by chemotherapy and radiation, and for which they are still receiving hormonal therapy. Here is an example to consider, but certainly modify it to meet your interests, activity level, and access to gyms or equipment.

Example Exercise Plan – Breast Cancer

55 year old woman who finished surgery a year ago, chemotherapy 6 months ago and radiation 3 months ago and recently started hormonal therapy with some mild increased hot flashes and already notices 10 pounds of weight gain above her normal. She still works full time.

Weekly Exercise Plan

> *Monday* – walk 20 minutes; stretch upper body

> *Tuesday* – walk 20 minutes; balance and resistance training; stretch upper body and lower body

> *Wednesday* – walk 20 minutes; stretch upper body

> *Thursday* – walk 20 minutes; balance and resistance training; stretch upper body and lower body

> *Friday* – walk 20 minutes; stretch upper body

> *Saturday* – walk 45 minutes with her friend; stretch upper body and lower body

> *Sunday* – walk 20 minutes; stretch upper body

Weekly Reminders:

✓ Incorporate daily stretching of her upper body to improve upper arm mobility and prevent and improve lymphedema. Lower body stretching should be done at least 3 times weekly.

✓ Plan to do daily aerobic exercise to improve her hot flashes and lose weight. Goal heart rate is 60-70% of maximum heart rate for at least 15 minutes to help burn fat and maintain a normal weight.

✓ Goal of 150 minutes of moderate intensity exercise per week.

✓ Incorporate resistance and strengthening at least 2 times per week on non-consecutive days to strengthen muscles and bones and prevent fractures. Since she is under 65 years old, she should plan to do 8-10 different exercises that target all the major muscle groups, performing 8-12 repetitions of each exercise. (If she was over 65 years old, then she should do lighter weights or less resistance and increase the repetitions to 10-15.)

✓ Incorporate flexibility and balance exercises, such as walking on uneven ground, 1 to 2 times per week to help prevent falls.

✓ Wear sunscreen if in the sun for more than 10 minutes since she completed chemotherapy and radiation treatments less than a year ago.

Daily Routine

Monday, Wednesday and Friday
- walk 20 minutes with a goal heart rate of 99-115 (60-70% maximum target heart rate)
- stretch upper body
  - neck roll
  - upper shoulder stretch
  - triceps stretch
  - shoulder and chest stretch

Tuesday and Thursday
- walk 20 minutes with a goal heart rate of 99-115 (60-70% maximum target heart rate)
- resistance training using body weight exercises except biceps (8-12 reps in 2-4 sets of each)
  - low plank
  - push-ups
  - swimmers
  - flying
  - arm circles
  - biceps using 5 pound free weights
  - triceps dips
  - reverse crunches
  - wall sits
  - lunges (also covers balance)
- stretch upper body
  - neck roll
  - upper shoulder stretch
  - triceps stretch
  - shoulder and chest stretch

- stretch lower body
  - low back/hips/hamstrings/glutes
  - hip flexors/quadriceps/back/calf (also covers balance)

Saturday

- walk 45 minutes with a friend; goal heart rate of 99-115 (60-70% maximum target heart rate)
- stretch upper body
  - neck roll
  - upper shoulder stretch
  - triceps stretch
  - shoulder and chest stretch
  - stretch lower body
  - low back/hips/hamstrings/glutes stretch
  - hip flexors/quadriceps/back/calf stretch (also covers balance)

Sunday

- walk 20 minutes with a goal heart rate of 99-115 (60-70% maximum target heart rate)
- stretch upper body
  - neck roll
  - upper shoulder stretch
  - triceps stretch
  - shoulder and chest stretch

Daily Reminders:

✓ Warm up and cool down for 2-5 minutes each day around exercises.

✓ Hold the stretches for 30 seconds. (If over 65 years old, then for 60 seconds.)

✓ Repeat each stretch at least twice and up to 4 times for each side.

✓ For resistance exercises, chose strengthening exercises that will work all the different major muscle groups. Plan a total of 8-10 exercises. Repeat each exercise 2-4 times (sets) for each side. In each set, perform 8-12 repetitions. (If over 65 years old, then perform 10-15 reps using lighter weights.)

✓ Maximum heart rate is 220 minus your age. Target heart rate during exercise is your maximum heart rate multiplied by 0.5 and by 0.85 which will give you the target range of 50-85% of your maximum heart rate. Fat burning typically happens at 60-70% maximum heart rate which is your maximum heart rate multiplied by 0.6 and 0.7 to get a range. Weight loss can occur when you reach your fat burning heart rate for at least 15 minutes.

✓ Directions of how to do the individual stretches can be found in the Flexibility Chapter.

✓ Directions for how to do the individual resistance exercises can be found in the Resistance and Strengthening Chapter.

CHAPTER 13
PROSTATE CANCER

Exercise can improve recovery from prostate cancer treatments, improve the tolerability of the treatments and lower the risk of developing a new or recurrent prostate cancer. As previously outlined in this book, exercise improves health and wellbeing in numerous ways which can lower the risk of cancer, including prostate cancer, and can help both recover from and tolerate the treatments for prostate cancer such as surgery, radiation, hormonal therapy and rarely, when indicated, chemotherapy. Whether you have had prostate cancer and are recovering from or going through treatments, or whether you want to avoid prostate cancer altogether, exercise should be an important part of your daily routine. Prostate cancer is fairly common, affecting about 1 in 8 men in their lifetime although the average age of diagnosis is closer to 70 years old. Prostate cancer treatments can affect men in many ways depending on the treatments received. Some people only require surgery, but others require radiation and/or hormonal therapies. Much less often, chemotherapy is also required for treatment of prostate cancer. Then there are the men who are focused on preventing prostate cancer altogether. This chapter will go into more detail on how exercise can specifically prevent prostate cancer, and how it benefits those recovering from treatments for prostate cancer, going through treatments for prostate cancer, or living with prostate cancer. For those who have received treatments for prostate cancer, there are considerations when exercising that will be outlined in this chapter. At the end of the chapter, I will outline an example work out plan for someone who has previously received prostate cancer treatments.

After what you have read so far in this book, if you are still wondering how exercise can prevent prostate cancer, then let's cover some of the specifics again. Research has shown that men who exercise regularly have lower rates of prostate cancer occurrences and recurrences. In addition, there are slightly higher rates of prostate cancer in men with diabetes, and exercise has been shown to lower the rates of diabetes and control blood sugar better in those who have diabetes. There is also an association with worse outcomes in men with prostate cancer who are obese, and exercise can lower the rates of obesity. When looking at the types of exercise that are beneficial, most types seem to be beneficial, but those focused on maintaining a normal weight seem to offer the most benefit at preventing prostate cancer.

Prostate cancer is a hormonally driven cancer, driven primarily by testosterone. Because of that, a lot of the treatments for prostate cancer are aimed at lowering levels of testosterone. This can create earlier than average menopause symptoms in men, including hot flashes, mood alterations, muscle weakness and atrophy, weaker bones, and weight gain, especially central obesity. When you start thinking about the hormonal effects of exercise on your body as we discussed in Section 1 of this book, it can start to make sense how exercise can not only prevent cancer, but can also help with the side effects of treatments. Insulin-like growth factor very likely plays an important role in the prevention of prostate cancer and is lowered with any type of exercise from aerobic activities to stretching and strengthening exercises, thereby potentially inhibiting cancer cell development. Other hormones including testosterone, growth hormone, thyroid hormone, epinephrine and insulin are involved with strengthening muscles and joints, managing the body's metabolism, and maintaining appropriate weight. You might wonder if the testosterone produced during exercise may be bad for prostate cancer, but it is a shorter surge during vigorous activities that actually helps during that short period of time to strengthen the muscles and joints, but doesn't significantly linger in the body to stimulate prostate cancer. Together, the hormones produced during exercise promote wellness of the body and likely all contribute to the lower rates of prostate cancer.

Other hormones that are produced during exercise called endorphins are also increased in the blood of people who participate in vigorous exercise. Remember that these hormones are structurally similar to morphine and can activate opioid receptors in the brain and elsewhere to minimize pain which may be how they improve arthritis pain and scar tissue pain. In addition, exercise can improve and prevent pain by strengthening the muscles that support the joints putting less stress on those joints. During hormonal treatments for prostate cancer, men have weaker bones from the chronic decreased testosterone which puts them at a higher risk of fractures. The hormones stimulated during exercise can reduce those fracture risks by strengthening the supporting muscles and joints around the bones. Recall also that exercise helps improve coordination and flexibility of the body which can lower the risk of falls. Better body mechanics promote health, lower injuries, and improve and prevent pain.

So keeping all this in consideration when thinking about types of exercises to incorporate into your routine helps come up with a successful program which should include aerobic endurance exercises, resistance or strength training and stretching. Balance exercises can be incorporated into some of the activities to simplify your routine. The aerobic exercises should be aimed at attaining and maintaining a normal weight. Now for some other considerations as you develop your routine.

For those who have undergone treatment for prostate cancer, there are certain muscle group exercises that are important to improve recovery and long-term wellbeing. Surgery can leave lasting physical changes including scar tissue which can cause leakage of urine. Radiation given to the pelvis can sometimes cause chronic loose stools or even diarrhea. This can easily lead to dehydration if you are not careful. You should avoid abdominal or pelvic floor exercises until you have healed enough from surgery. Since different surgeries can have different recovery rates, check with your surgeon as to when you could start an exercise program that might cause jarring or stress to the abdomen and pelvis. Once you start the lower body exercises, start slow and proceed as your body is ready so that you do not delay healing. However, pelvic floor exercises are very important to improving urinary continence and providing long term good quality of life, so these are important exercise to have in your daily routine.

Hormonal therapy treatments if indicated to treat your prostate cancer can create male menopausal symptoms such as hot flashes, irritability, depression, fatigue, and sometimes cause weaker bones while you receive them. It may surprise you, but exercise has also been shown to improve menopausal symptoms such as hot flashes and arthritis pain associated with menopause. This is felt to be from the increased healthy and safe hormone production produced during exercising that we discussed above, as well as increased serotonin and norepinephrine during exercise which improves depression and anxiety, improves sleep, and offers a sense of wellbeing. Often regular daily aerobic exercise alone can manage menopausal symptoms without the need of additional supplements or medicines. Incorporating some strengthening, flexibility and balance exercises will help keep the bones strong and prevent falls and fractures. Often weight gain can be seen while on hormonal therapy treatments which can be countered by regular aerobic exercise focusing on keeping your target heart rate range in the 60% to 70% of your maximum heart rate range for at least 15 minutes per session where fat burning occurs.

If you are exercising while receiving chemotherapy, then it is important to know the side effects of the specific medicines you are receiving when considering your exercise routine. If the chemotherapy you are receiving can cause fatigue, weakness, or dizziness which all can occur with anemia, a common side effect of chemotherapy, then shorten your aerobic exercise that you do at any given time to smaller more frequent intervals at slower paces and make sure to hydrate well prior, during and after you exercise. In this situation, you may also need to do less weight or resistance when doing strengthening exercises. You can still stay toned by doing more repetitions of lighter weights during this time. If the chemotherapy you are receiving lowers your immune system, then be careful working out with crowds, like at gyms or in large groups. Most chemotherapy will make you more sensitive to the sun for at least 6 months and up to a year, so wear sunscreen when you are in the sun for more than about 10 to 15 minutes depending on your skin type. Fair complexions may require sunscreen for even a few minutes of sun exposure. Chemotherapy can cause dry skin and sometimes rashes; excessive sweating can worsen those conditions. Make sure to moisturize your skin. You may even need to do short intervals of aerobic exercise to minimize sweating until you have recovered from the chemotherapy.

So what might an exercise plan look like for a man who has received treatment for prostate cancer which included surgery or radiation, and for which they are still receiving hormonal therapy. Here is an example to consider, but certainly modify it to meet your interests, activity level, and access to gyms or equipment.

Example Exercise Plan – Prostate Cancer

70 year old man with prostate cancer surgically removed 5 years ago but experienced increasing PSA for which he is receiving hormonal therapy with shots periodically who has symptoms of mild hot flashes a few times a week, mild muscle weakness mostly in his arms and more weight gain around his stomach.

Weekly Exercise Plan

Monday – walk 30 minutes including 5 minutes stairs; stretch lower body

Tuesday –strength training; stretch lower body and upper body

Wednesday – walk 30 minutes including 5 minutes stairs; stretch lower body

Thursday –strength training; stretch lower body and upper body

Friday – walk 30 minutes including 5 minutes stairs; stretch lower body

Saturday – strength training; stretch lower body and upper body

Sunday – bike 60 minutes; stretch lower body

Weekly Reminders:

✓ Incorporate abdominal and pelvic floor exercises and stretching at least 5 times per week but preferably daily to maintain good urinary and bowel movement control.

✓ Plan to do aerobic exercise 4 days per week to maintain normal weight and improve hot flashes. Goal heart rate is 60-70% of maximum heart rate for at least 15 minutes to help burn fat and maintain a normal weight.

✓ Goal of 150 minutes of moderate intensity exercise per week.

✓ Incorporate resistance and strengthening at least 3 times per week on non-consecutive days to strengthen muscles and bones and prevent fractures. Since he is over 65 years old, he should plan to do 8-10 different exercises that target all the major muscle groups, performing 10-15 repetitions of each exercise. (If he was under 65 years old, then he should do heavier weights or more resistance and lower the repetitions to 8-12.)

✓ Incorporate flexibility and balance exercises, such as walking on uneven ground, 1 to 2 times per week to help prevent falls.

Daily Routine

Monday, Wednesday and Friday

• walk 30 minutes including 5 minutes stairs, goal heart rate of 90-105 (60-70% max heart rate)

    ○ stairs help with balance and lower body strengthening

• stretch lower body

    ○ low back/hips/hamstrings stretch

    ○ hip flexor and glute stretch

    ○ adductor leg stretch

Tuesday, Thursday and Saturday

- strength training (10-15 reps in 2-4 sets of each) using a combination of free weights and
    - machines at the gym
    - biceps curls
    - overhead press
    - standing row
    - dips
    - push-ups
    - high plank
    - plank shoulder taps
    - chest fly
    - wall sits
    - leg extension
    - prone leg curls
    - calf raises
    - reverse crunches
    - twists
    - hip raises
    - stretch lower body
    - low back/hips/hamstrings stretch
    - hip flexor and glute stretch
    - adductor leg stretch
    - stretch upper body
    - neck roll
    - upper shoulder stretch
    - triceps stretch
    - shoulder and chest stretch

Sunday

- bike 60 minutes, goal heart rate 90-105 (60-70% max heart rate)
- stretch lower body
  ◦ low back/hips/hamstrings stretch
  ◦ hip flexor and glute stretch
- adductor leg stretch

Daily Reminders:

✓ Warm up and cool down for 2-5 minutes each day around exercises.

✓ Hold the stretches for 60 seconds. (If under 65 years old, then hold the stretch for 30 seconds.)

✓ Repeat each stretch at least twice and up to 4 times for each side.

✓ For resistance exercises, chose strengthening exercises that will work all the different major muscle groups. Plan a total of 8-10 exercises. Repeat each exercise 2-4 times (sets) for each side. In each set, perform 10-15 repetitions using lighter weights or resistance. (If under 65 years old, then perform 8-12 reps using heavier weight or more resistance.)

✓ Maximum heart rate is 220 minus your age. Target heart rate during exercise is your maximum heart rate multiplied by 0.5 and by 0.85 which will give you the target range of 50-85% of your maximum heart rate. Fat burning typically happens at 60-70% maximum heart rate which is your maximum heart rate multiplied by 0.6 and 0.7 to get a range. Weight loss can occur when you reach your fat burning heart rate for at least 15 minutes.

✓ Directions of how to do the stretches can be found in the Flexibility Chapter.

✓ Directions for how to do the strength exercises can be found in the Resistance and Strengthening Chapter.

CHAPTER 14

GASTROINTESTINAL CANCER

Exercise can improve recovery from gastrointestinal cancer treatments, improve the tolerability of the treatments and lower the risk of developing a new or recurrent gastrointestinal cancer. Gastrointestinal cancers include any of the cancers that can affect the gastrointestinal system which include the more common colon and rectal cancers, but also the less common cancers of other organs along the gastrointestinal tract such as the esophagus, stomach, small bowel, pancreas, and bile ducts. As previously outlined in this book, exercise improves health and wellbeing in numerous ways which can lower the risk of cancer, including gastrointestinal cancers, and can help both recover from and tolerate the treatments for gastrointestinal cancers such as surgery, radiation, and chemotherapy. Whether you have had a gastrointestinal cancer and are recovering from or going through treatments, or whether you want to avoid developing a gastrointestinal cancer altogether, exercise should be an important part of your daily routine.

Gastrointestinal cancers are fairly common, with colon cancer being the second most common cancer in both women and men. The average age of diagnosis is between 65-70 years old for most gastrointestinal cancers. Surgery is very often a part of the treatment for gastrointestinal cancers. With colon cancer, surgery is usually one of the first treatments, but for other gastrointestinal cancers, surgery is often done after treatments with chemotherapy and radiation. Sometimes surgery is not needed at all. Many people diagnosed with gastrointestinal cancers will require chemotherapy and radiation which can be done together or separate depending on the cancer type. There are many people who are focused on preventing gastrointestinal cancers altogether. This chapter will go into more detail on how exercise can specifically prevent gastrointestinal cancers, and how it benefits those recovering from treatments for gastrointestinal cancer, going through treatments for a gastrointestinal cancer, or living with a gastrointestinal cancer. For those who have received treatments for gastrointestinal cancers, there are considerations when exercising that will be outlined in this chapter. At the end of the chapter, I will outline an example work out plan for someone who has previously received colon cancer treatments and someone who has received rectal cancer treatments as the symptoms from treatments and beneficial exercises can vary slightly.

Lower rates of gastrointestinal cancers occur in people who exercise regularly and maintain a normal weight. Research has shown that people who exercise regularly have lower rates of colorectal cancer occurrences and recurrences. In addition, there are slightly higher rates of colorectal, pancreas, and bile duct cancers in people with diabetes, and exercise has been shown to lower the rates of diabetes and control blood sugar better in those who have diabetes. There is also an association with worse outcomes in people with gastrointestinal cancers who are obese, and exercise can lower the rates of obesity. When looking at the types of exercise that are beneficial, most types seem to be beneficial, but those focused on maintaining a normal weight seem to offer the most benefit at preventing gastrointestinal cancers.

As has been previously discussed, there are a lot of hormones that are produced when we exercise and are active. These hormones

work in different ways to prevent cancer occurrences and recurrences. When considering gastrointestinal cancers, insulin-like growth
factor is likely one of the more important hormones which can be
lowered during all types of activities potentially inhibiting cancer cell
development. Other hormones including growth hormone, thyroid
hormone, epinephrine, insulin, and testosterone are involved with
managing the body's metabolism, maintaining appropriate weight,
and strengthening muscles and joints. Together, the hormones produced during exercise promote wellness of the body and likely all
contribute to the lower rates of gastrointestinal cancers.

Other hormones produced during exercise called endorphins are
also increased in the blood of people who participate in moderate
to vigorous exercise. Remember that these hormones are structurally
similar to morphine and can activate opioid receptors in the brain
and elsewhere to minimize pain which may be how they improve
arthritis pain and scar tissue pain. In addition, exercise can improve
and prevent pain by strengthening the muscles that support the
joints putting less stress on those joints. Recall also that exercise helps
improve coordination and flexibility of the body which can lower the
risk of falls. Better body mechanics promote health, lower injuries,
and improve and prevent pain.

So keeping all these healthy benefits of exercise in consideration
when planning the types of exercises to incorporate into your routine helps come up with a successful program which should include
aerobic endurance exercises, resistance or strength training and
stretching. Balance exercises can be incorporated into some of the
activities to simplify your routine. The aerobic exercises should be
aimed at attaining and maintaining a normal weight.

For those who have undergone treatment for a gastrointestinal cancer, there are certain muscle group exercises that are important to improve recovery and long-term wellbeing. Surgery can leave lasting physical changes including scar tissue, ostomy bags, and sometimes chronic pain. Radiation given to the abdomen or pelvis can sometimes cause chronic loose stools or even diarrhea and can sometimes make scar tissue worse. Dehydration can occur easily if you have chronic diarrhea or if you suffer from difficulty with swallowing after surgery for esophagus or stomach cancers. You should avoid abdominal or pelvic floor exercises until you have healed enough from surgery. Since different surgeries can have different recovery rates, check with your surgeon as to when you could start an exercise program that might cause jarring or stress to the abdomen and pelvis. Once you start the abdomen and lower body exercises, start slowly and proceed as your body is ready so that you do not delay healing. You may need to get an abdominal binder or at least wear a tight undergarment during exercises that prevent hernias from developing after abdominal surgeries. If you have an ostomy bag, consider doing abdominal exercises that are strengthening your back muscles more than exercises that are focused on the front abdominal muscles to avoid hernias. However, abdominal and pelvic floor exercises are very important to controlling pain from scar tissue and providing long term good quality of life, so these are important exercises to have in your daily routine.

If you are exercising while receiving chemotherapy, then it is important to know the side effects of the specific medicines you are receiving when considering your exercise routine. If the chemotherapy you are receiving can cause fatigue, weakness, or dizziness which can also occur with anemia, then shorten your aerobic exercise that you do at any given time to shorter more frequent intervals at slower paces and make sure to hydrate well prior to, during and after you exercise. In this situation, you may also need to do less weight or resistance when doing strengthening exercises. You can still stay toned by doing more repetitions of lighter weights during this time. If the chemotherapy you are receiving lowers your immune system, then be careful working out with crowds, like at gyms or in large groups.

Not only does surgery and radiation for gastrointestinal cancers lead to bowel changes like constipation and diarrhea, but chemotherapy can compound these symptoms or change the symptoms. Sometimes, nausea or vomiting can occur, or the liquids and foods that you take in have to be modified due to side effects from the treatments. Staying well hydrated will help with these side effects. Try to hydrate just before and after exercising, but avoid eating within about 45 to 60 minutes prior to and after exercising to help with these symptoms during your exercise routine. Often exercise will actually make these side effects better. There are some types of chemotherapy given for gastrointestinal cancers that can cause numbness and tingling in the hands or feet. Being careful with balance exercises during this time is important, but exercise can actually often improve these symptoms as well. There is also a chemotherapy medicine often given for colon and rectal cancers that will cause sensitivity to the cold. If you are exercising in the cold weather, be sure to wear gloves and a hat. Sometimes it is actually better to avoid aerobic exercise the few days after receiving the chemotherapy since it can cause more shortness of breath, cough and wheezing in those with respiratory diseases like asthma. Most chemotherapy will make you more sensitive to the sun for at least 6 months and up to a year, so wear sunscreen when you are in the sun for more than about 10 to 15 minutes depending on your skin type. Fair complexions may require sunscreen for even a few minutes of sun exposure. Chemotherapy can cause dry skin and sometimes rashes; excessive sweating can worsen those conditions. Make sure to moisturize your skin and you may need to do short intervals of aerobic exercise to minimize sweating while on chemotherapy.

People diagnosed with gastrointestinal cancers and undergoing treatments can develop symptoms that affect well-being in other ways. Exercise can improve the sense of well-being by increasing levels of serotonin and norepinephrine during exercise which improves depression and anxiety, and can improve sleep. Incorporating some strengthening, flexibility and balance exercises will help keep the bones strong and prevent falls and fractures. Often weight gain can occur after surgery and chemotherapy which can be countered by regular aerobic exercise focusing on keeping your target heart rate range in the 60% to 70% of your maximum heart rate range for at least 15 minutes per session where fat burning occurs.

So what might an exercise plan look like for someone who has received treatment for rectal cancer or is undergoing treatment for colon cancer. Here are some examples to consider, but certainly modify it to meet your interests, activity level, and access to gyms or equipment.

Example Exercise Plan – Rectal Cancer

65 year old man with rectal cancer treated with chemotherapy and radiation followed by surgery that required a colostomy now 3 years out from treatment. He is struggling with weight gain from lack of activity after all of his treatments.

Weekly Exercise Plan

Monday – walk 30 minutes including 5 minutes stairs; stretch lower body

Tuesday –strength training; stretch lower body and upper body

Wednesday – walk 30 minutes including 5 minutes stairs; stretch lower body

Thursday –strength training; stretch lower body and upper body

Friday – walk 30 minutes including 5 minutes stairs; stretch lower body

Saturday – strength training; stretch lower body and upper body

Sunday – bike 60 minutes; stretch lower body

Weekly Reminders:
- ✓ Incorporate abdominal and pelvic floor stretching at least 5 times per week but preferably daily to maintain good urinary control.
- ✓ Abdominal exercises will focus more on back strengthening since he has an ostomy bag.
- ✓ Plan to do aerobic exercise 4 days per week to maintain normal weight. Goal heart rate is 60-70% of maximum heart rate for at least 15 minutes to help burn fat and maintain a normal weight.
- ✓ Goal of 150 minutes of moderate intensity exercise per week.
- ✓ Incorporate resistance and strengthening at least 3 times per week on non-consecutive days to strengthen muscles and bones and prevent fractures. Since he is over 65 years old, he should plan to do 8-10 different exercises that target all the major muscle groups, performing 10-15 repetitions of each exercise. (If

he was under 65 years old, then he should do heavier weights or more resistance and lower the repetitions to 8-12.)

✓ Incorporate flexibility and balance exercises, such as walking on uneven ground, 1 to 2 times per week to help prevent falls.

Daily Routine

Monday, Wednesday and Friday

- walk 30 minutes including 5 minutes stairs, goal heart rate of 93-108 (60-70% max heart rate)
  - ○ stairs help with balance and lower body strengthening
- stretch lower body
  - ○ low back/hips/hamstrings stretch
  - ○ hip flexor and glute stretch
  - ○ adductor leg stretch

Tuesday, Thursday and Saturday

- strength training (10-15 reps in 2-4 sets of each) using resistance bands at home
  - ○ biceps curls
  - ○ overhead press
  - ○ standing row
  - ○ dips
  - ○ trunk rotations
  - ○ low to high trunk rotations
  - ○ side bend
  - ○ twists
  - ○ chest fly
  - ○ front squats
  - ○ standing adduction quadriceps
  - ○ standing abduction quadriceps

- ○ calf raises

- stretch lower body
  - ○ low back/hips/hamstrings stretch
  - ○ hip flexor and glute stretch
  - ○ adductor leg stretch

- stretch upper body
  - ○ neck roll
  - ○ upper shoulder stretch
  - ○ triceps stretch
  - ○ shoulder and chest stretch

Sunday

- bike 60 minutes, goal heart rate 93-108 (60-70% max heart rate)
- stretch lower body
  - ○ low back/hips/hamstrings stretch
  - ○ hip flexor and glute stretch
  - ○ adductor leg stretch

Daily Reminders:

- ✓ Warm up and cool down for 2-5 minutes each day around exercises.
- ✓ Hold the stretches for 60 seconds. (If under 65 years old, then hold the stretch for 30 seconds.)
- ✓ Repeat each stretch at least twice and up to 4 times for each side.
- ✓ For resistance exercises, chose strengthening exercises that will work all the different major muscle groups. Plan at least 8-10 different exercises. Repeat each exercise 2-4 times (sets) for each side. In each set, perform 10-15 repetitions. (If under 65 years

old, then decrease the reps to 8-12 and use heavier weights or more resistance.)

✓ Maximum heart rate is 220 minus your age. Target heart rate during exercise is your maximum heart rate multiplied by 0.5 and by 0.85 which will give you the target range of 50-85% of your maximum heart rate. Fat burning typically happens at 60-70% maximum heart rate which is your maximum heart rate multiplied by 0.6 and 0.7 to get a range. Weight loss can occur when you reach your fat burning heart rate for at least 15 minutes.

✓ Directions of how to do the stretches can be found in the Flexibility Chapter.

✓ Directions for how to do the strength exercises can be found in the Resistance and Strengthening Chapter.

Example Exercise Plan – Colon Cancer

60 year old woman with colon cancer treated with surgery and currently receiving chemotherapy for prevention of recurrence. She is having neuropathy from the chemotherapy which is numbness in her fingertips and feet that is worsened by cold.

Weekly Exercise Plan – while receiving chemotherapy

Monday – walk 10 minutes twice a day; lower body strength training; stretch lower body

Tuesday –walk 10 minutes twice a day; upper body strength training; stretch lower/upper body

Wednesday – walk 10 minutes twice a day; lower body strengthening; stretch lower body

Thursday –walk 10 minutes twice a day; upper body strength training; stretch lower/upper body

Friday – walk 10 minutes twice a day; lower body strengthening; stretch lower body

Saturday – walk 10 minutes twice a day; upper body strength training; stretch lower/upper body

Sunday – walk 15 minutes twice a day; stretch lower body

Weekly Exercise Plan – after chemotherapy is complete and energy is improving

Monday – walk 15 minutes twice a day; stretch lower body

Tuesday – strength training lower/upper body; stretch lower/upper body

Wednesday – walk 15 minutes twice a day; stretch lower body

Thursday – strength training lower/upper body; stretch lower/upper body

Friday – walk 15 minutes twice a day; stretch lower body

Saturday – strength training lower/upper body; stretch lower/upper body

Sunday – walk 30 minutes twice a day; stretch lower body

Weekly Exercise Plan – about 6 months after chemotherapy completed

Monday – walk 35 minutes once a day; stretch lower body

Tuesday – strength training lower/upper body; stretch lower/upper body

Wednesday – walk 35 minutes once a day; stretch lower body

Thursday – strength training lower/upper body; stretch lower/ upper body

Friday – walk 35 minutes once a day; stretch lower body

Saturday – strength training lower/upper body; stretch lower/ upper body

Sunday – walk 45 minutes once a day; stretch lower body

Weekly Reminders:

- ✓ Incorporate abdominal stretching at least 5 times per week but preferably daily.
- ✓ Plan to do daily aerobic exercise. While she is on chemotherapy, shorter intervals will work better for her and weight loss is not a goal so her heart rate goal should be 50% of maximum, lower target range. When she finishes chemotherapy, then she should have a goal heart rate of 60-70% of her maximum heart rate for at least 15 minutes to help burn fat and maintain a normal weight.
- ✓ Goal of 150 minutes of aerobic exercise per week.
- ✓ Incorporate resistance and strengthening at least 3 times per week on non-consecutive days to strengthen muscles and bones and prevent fractures. Since she is under 65 years old, she should plan to do 8-10 different exercises that target all the major muscle groups, performing 8-12 repetitions of each exercise. While on chemotherapy, she may plan to do lower weights for 10-15 reps. (If she was over 65 years old, then she should do lighter weights or less resistance and increase the repetitions to 10-15.)

✓ Incorporate flexibility and balance exercises, such as walking on uneven ground, 1 to 2 times per week to help prevent falls.

✓ Wear sunscreen if in the sun for more than 10 minutes since she is on chemotherapy and she should continue to wear sunscreen until at least one year after completion of chemotherapy.

✓ While she is on active chemotherapy, she needs to take precautions. Her chemotherapy can lower her immune system so it would be preferable for her to minimize crowded gyms. Also, she may develop anemia which may cause more fatigue. This is a good time to split her exercises into shorter intervals to prevent overwhelming fatigue. She may have worse constipation or diarrhea from the chemotherapy and should hydrate well throughout the day and especially around her exercises to improve those symptoms and prevent dehydration. Because of her symptoms of neuropathy, she should wear gloves if it is cold outside and wear good shoes with all of her exercises to protect her feet.

Daily Routine – while receiving chemotherapy

Monday, Wednesday and Friday
- walk 10 minutes in the morning and 10 minutes in the evening
- strength training lower body
    - wall sits
    - lunges
    - calf raises
- stretch lower body
    - hamstring stretch
    - quadriceps stretch
    - adductor leg stretch
    - hip flexor and glute stretch

- low back stretch

Tuesday, Thursday and Saturday
- walk 10 minutes in the morning and 10 minutes in the evening
- strength training upper body
  - wall plank
  - arm circles
  - bicep curls
  - dips
- stretch upper body
  - neck roll
  - upper shoulder stretch
  - triceps stretch
  - shoulder and chest stretch
- stretch lower body
  - hamstring stretch
  - quadriceps stretch
  - adductor leg stretch
  - hip flexor and glute stretch
  - low back stretch

Sunday
- walk 15 minutes in the morning and 15 minutes in the evening
- stretch lower body
  - hamstring stretch
  - quadriceps stretch
  - adductor leg stretch
  - hip flexor and glute stretch
  - low back stretch

Weekly Exercise Plan – about 6 months after chemotherapy completed

Monday, Wednesday and Friday
- walk 35 minutes once a day including 5 minutes stairs,
    - goal heart rate of 96-112 (60-70% max heart rate)
    - stairs help with balance and lower body strengthening
- stretch lower body
    - hamstring stretch
    - quadriceps stretch
    - adductor leg stretch
    - hip flexor and glute stretch
    - low back stretch

Tuesday, Thursday and Saturday
- strength training lower and upper body
    - high plank
    - plank shoulder taps
    - side plank body rotations
    - squats
    - lunges
    - arm circles with weights
    - bicep curls with weights
    - dips
    - twists
    - leg lifts
- stretch lower body
    - hamstring stretch
    - quadriceps stretch
    - adductor leg stretch
    - hip flexor and glute stretch
    - low back stretch
- stretch upper body
    - neck roll

- upper shoulder stretch
- triceps stretch
- shoulder and chest stretch

Sunday

- walk 45 minutes once a day including 5 minutes stairs,
  - goal heart rate of 96-112 (60-70% max heart rate)
  - stretch lower body
  - hamstring stretch
  - quadriceps stretch
  - adductor leg stretch
  - hip flexor and glute stretch
  - low back stretch

Daily Reminders

✓ Warm up and cool down for 2-5 minutes each day around exercises.

✓ Hold the stretches for 30 seconds. (If over 65 years old, then hold the stretch for 60 seconds.)

✓ Repeat each stretch at least twice and up to 4 times for each side.

✓ For resistance exercises, chose strengthening exercises that will work all the different major muscle groups. Plan at least 8-10 exercises. Repeat each exercise 2-4 times (sets) for each side. In each set, perform 8-12 repetitions. She may decide to do lighter weights while on chemotherapy for 10-15 reps. (If she was over 65 years old, then perform 10-15 reps using lighter weights.)

✓ Wear sunscreen if in the sun for more than 10 minutes since on chemotherapy and continue to wear sunscreen until at least one year after completion of chemotherapy.

✓ While she is on active chemotherapy, she needs to take precautions. Minimize crowded gyms while on chemotherapy given lowered immune system. Split exercises into shorter intervals while on chemotherapy to prevent overwhelming fatigue. Stay well hydrated. Wear gloves if it is cold outside and wear good shoes with all of her exercises to protect her feet.

✓ Maximum heart rate is 220 minus your age. Target heart rate during exercise is your maximum heart rate multiplied by 0.5 and by 0.85 which will give you the target range of 50-85% of your maximum heart rate. Fat burning typically happens at 60-70% maximum heart rate which is your maximum heart rate multiplied by 0.6 and 0.7 to get a range. Weight loss can occur when you reach your fat burning heart rate for at least 15 minutes. About 6 months after completion of chemotherapy, it is reasonable to try to reach the fat burning heart rate of 60-70% during exercise. Until then, while on chemotherapy and shortly after finishing chemotherapy, focus on staying active but not overdoing it.

✓ Strength training will be done with body resistance exercises primarily.

✓ Directions of how to do the stretches can be found in the Flexibility Chapter.

✓ Directions for how to do the strength exercises can be found in the Resistance and Strengthening Chapter.

CHAPTER 15
LUNG CANCER

Exercise can improve recovery from lung cancer treatments, improve the tolerability of the treatments and lower the risk of developing a new or recurrent lung cancer. As previously outlined in this book, exercise improves health and wellbeing in numerous ways which can lower the risk of cancer, including lung cancer, and can help both recover from and tolerate the treatments for lung cancer including surgery, radiation, and chemotherapy. Whether you have had lung cancer and are recovering from or going through treatments, or whether you want to avoid lung cancer altogether, exercise should be an important part of your daily routine. Lung cancer treatments can affect people in many ways depending on the treatments received. Some people only require surgery, but others require radiation and/or chemotherapy. There are also people focused on preventing lung cancer altogether. This chapter will go into more detail on how exercise can benefit those recovering from treatments for lung cancer, going through treatments for lung cancer, living with lung cancer, or just trying to prevent it altogether. For those who have received treatments for lung cancer, there are considerations when exercising that will be outlined in this chapter. At the end of the chapter, I will outline an example work out plan for someone recovering from lung cancer treatments.

Exercise plays an important role for people recovering from lung cancer treatments, and can likely also prevent occurrences and recurrences of lung cancer. Environmental exposures such as cigarette smoke still pose some of the highest risks leading to lung cancer, so decreasing cigarette smoke exposure is very important. Those people who participate in at least 150 minutes of moderate exercise per week are less likely to smoke as much as those who do not exercise. In addition, diabetes has been linked to worse outcomes in people with lung cancer undergoing treatments. Exercise has been shown to lower the rates of diabetes and control blood sugar better in those who have diabetes.

Exercise also causes changes in the hormone levels of the body which can lower the risk of lung cancer and improve tolerability and recovery from treatments for lung cancer. Insulin-like growth factor very likely plays an important role in lung cancer and is lowered with any type of activity, even stretching, which can potentially inhibit cancer cell development. Other hormones including growth hormone, thyroid hormone, epinephrine, insulin and testosterone are involved with strengthening muscles and joints, managing the body's metabolism, and maintaining appropriate weight. Together, these hormones produced during exercise promote wellness of the body and likely all contribute to the lower rates of lung cancer and improved tolerability of lung cancer treatments. Endorphins are hormones increased in the blood of people who participate in vigorous exercise. Remember that these hormones are structurally similar to morphine and can activate opioid receptors in the brain and elsewhere to minimize pain which may be how they improve arthritis pain and scar tissue pain. In addition, exercise can improve and prevent pain by strengthening the muscles that support the joints putting less stress on those joints. Risks of fractures are reduced by having stronger muscles and healthier joints. Recall also that exercise helps improve coordination and flexibility of the body which can lower the risk of falls. Better body mechanics promote health, lower injuries, and improve and prevent pain. Finally, exercise can improve the sense of well-being by increasing levels of serotonin and norepinephrine during exercise which improves depression and anxiety, and can improve sleep.

For those who have undergone treatment for lung cancer, there are certain exercises that are important to improve recovery and long-term wellbeing. Surgery can leave lasting physical changes including scar tissue which can cause tightness of the skin and back joints, and more limited breathing due to loss of lung tissue. Radiation can also lead to similar breathing changes. As you recover from surgery, the surgeon will release you to start increasing your activity usually around 4-6 weeks after surgery. Sometimes they will recommend something called pulmonary rehab to help you improve your breathing. Once you start upper body exercises, start slow and proceed as your body is ready so that you do not cause the surgical incision site to heal more slowly. In addition, radiation may slow your ability to progress with your exercises during the treatments. The radiation can cause tightness of the skin and local tissues, and it can take 6 to 12 months, even sometimes longer, for that tightness to resolve. Stretching your upper body which includes your arm, shoulder, back and chest will be important in your exercise routine and should be done at least 4-5 days per week, and I would suggest daily. Find a time to set aside to do them as part of your daily routine so that you do not forget such as when you take your shower or just prior to going to bed. Also, remember to use sun screen when you are in the sun for up to 12 months after radiation or chemotherapy as your skin is more sensitive to the sun.

If you are exercising while receiving chemotherapy, then it is important to know the side effects of the specific medicines you are

receiving when considering your exercise routine. If the chemotherapy you are receiving can cause fatigue, weakness, or dizziness
which all can occur with anemia, then shorten your aerobic exercise that you do at any given time to shorter more frequent intervals at slower paces and make sure to hydrate well prior to, during
and after you exercise. In this situation, you may also need to do less
weight or resistance when doing strengthening exercises. You can
still stay toned by doing more repetitions of lighter weights during this
time. If the chemotherapy you are receiving lowers your immune
system, then be careful working out with crowds, like at gyms or in
large groups. Chemotherapy often leads to bowel changes such as
constipation or diarrhea, and sometimes nausea and even vomiting.
Staying well hydrated will help with these side effects. Often exercise
will actually make these side effects better. There are some types
of chemotherapy given for lung cancer that can cause numbness
and tingling in the hands or feet. Being careful with balance exercises during this time is important, but exercise can actually often
improve these symptoms as well. Most chemotherapy will make you
more sensitive to the sun for at least 6 months and up to a year, so
wear sunscreen when you are in the sun for more than about 10 to 15
minutes depending on your skin type. Fair complexions may require
sunscreen for even a few minutes of sun exposure. Chemotherapy
can cause dry skin and sometimes rashes; excessive sweating can
worsen those conditions. Make sure to moisturize your skin and you
may need to do short intervals of aerobic exercise to minimize sweating until the side effects of chemotherapy are gone.

So when considering the effects of lung cancer treatments, modifying the types of exercises to incorporate into your routine helps you
to come up with a successful exercise program which should include
aerobic endurance exercises, resistance or strength training and

stretching. Balance exercises can be incorporated into some of the activities to simplify your routine. Here is an example of an exercise plan for someone recovering from lung cancer treatment. This is just an example; certainly modify it to meet your interests, activity level, and access to gyms or equipment.

Example Exercise Plan – Lung Cancer

70 year old man was diagnosed with lung cancer 9 months ago and had surgery followed by chemotherapy. He is still struggling with shortness of breath with activities and fatigue.

Weekly Exercise Plan – beginning

Monday – walk 20 minutes; strength training; stretch upper body and lower body

Tuesday – walk 20 minutes; deep breathing exercises; stretch upper body

Wednesday – walk 20 minutes; strength training; stretch upper body and lower body

Thursday – walk 20 minutes; deep breathing exercises; stretch upper body

Friday – walk 20 minutes; strength training; stretch upper body and lower body

Saturday – walk 20 minutes; deep breathing exercises; stretch upper body

Sunday – walk 20 minutes; deep breathing exercises; stretch upper body

Weekly Exercise Plan – after 6 months of increasing walking time

Monday – walk 20 minutes; strength training; stretch upper body and lower body

Tuesday – walk 45 minutes; stretch upper body

Wednesday – walk 20 minutes; strength training; stretch upper body and lower body

Thursday – walk 45 minutes; stretch upper body

Friday – walk 20 minutes; strength training; stretch upper body and lower body

Saturday – walk 45 minutes; stretch upper body

Sunday – walk 45 minutes; stretch upper body

Weekly Reminders:

✓ Incorporate daily stretching of his upper body at a minimum to improve surgical incision pain.

✓ Plan to do daily aerobic exercise to improve breathing with short bursts of faster walking.

✓ Goal of 150 minutes of moderate intensity exercise per week.

✓ Incorporate resistance and strengthening at least 3 times per week on non-consecutive days to strengthen muscles and bones and prevent fractures. Since he is over 65 years old, he should plan to do 8-10 different exercises that target all the major muscle groups, performing 10-15 repetitions of each exercise. (If he was under 65 years old, then he should do heavier weights or more resistance and decrease the repetitions to 8-12.)

✓ Incorporate flexibility and balance exercises, such as walking on uneven ground, 1 to 2 times per week to help prevent falls.

✓ Wear sunscreen if in the sun for more than 10 minutes since he completed chemotherapy treatments less than a year ago. (Same would be true if he had completed radiation during this time.)

✓ When recovering from lung surgery, it is important to get lung volumes back which can be improved with deep breathing exercises, such is blowing up balloons or singing.

Daily Routine – beginning

Week at a glance ~ to start with

Monday, Wednesday and Friday
- walk 20 minutes,
  - goal heart rate 75-127 (50-85% of max heart rate)
- strength training with a resistance band
  - push-ups
  - chest press
  - chest fly
  - pull-aparts
  - standing row
  - forward raise
  - wood choppers
  - trunk rotation
  - bicep curls
  - wall sits
- stretch upper body and lower body
  - neck roll
  - upper shoulder
  - triceps
  - shoulder and chest

- o   low back
- o   hip flexor and glute

Tuesday, Thursday, Saturday and Sunday

- walk 20 minutes
  - o   goal heart rate 75-127 (50-85% of max heart rate)
- deep breathing exercises
  - o   blow up 5-10 standard balloons
- stretch upper body
  - o   neck roll
  - o   upper shoulder
  - o   triceps
  - o   shoulder and chest

Daily Routine – after 6 months of increasing walking time

Monday, Wednesday and Friday

- walk 20 minutes,
- goal heart rate 75-127 (50-85% of max heart rate)
- strength training with a resistance band
  - o   push-ups
  - o   chest press
  - o   chest fly
  - o   pull-aparts
  - o   standing row
  - o   forward raise
  - o   wood choppers
  - o   trunk rotation
  - o   bicep curls
  - o   wall sits
- stretch upper body and lower body
  - o   neck roll

- upper shoulder
- triceps
- shoulder and chest
- low back
- hip flexor and glute

Tuesday, Thursday, Saturday and Sunday

- walk 45 minutes total, goal heart rate 75-127 (50-85% of max heart rate), 15 minutes at the lower heart rate goal, then speed up for 5 minutes to get your heart rate at the higher goal level, then 15 minutes at the lower goal, then 5 minutes at the higher goal, then 15 minutes at the lower goal, and then end with 5 minutes at the higher goal.
- stretch upper body
  - neck roll
  - upper shoulder
  - triceps
  - shoulder and chest

Daily Reminders:

- ✓ Warm up and cool down for 2-5 minutes each day around exercises.
- ✓ Hold the stretches for 60 seconds. (If under 65 years old, then for 30 seconds.)
- ✓ Repeat each stretch at least twice and up to 4 times for each side.
- ✓ For strength exercises, chose exercises that will work all the different major muscle groups. Plan a total of 8-10 exercises. Repeat each exercise 2-4 times (sets) for each side. In each set, perform 10-15 repetitions. (If he was under 65 years old, then he

should do heavier weights or more resistance and decrease the repetitions to 8-12.)

✓ Maximum heart rate is 220 minus your age. Target heart rate during exercise is your maximum heart rate multiplied by 0.5 and by 0.85 which will give you the target range of 50-85% of your maximum heart rate. Fat burning typically happens at 60-70% maximum heart rate which is your maximum heart rate multiplied by 0.6 and 0.7 to get a range. Weight loss can occur when you reach your fat burning heart rate for at least 15 minutes.

✓ When recovering from lung surgery, it is important to improve lung volumes by working on deep breathing exercises, such is blowing up balloons, singing, or simply working on short time periods of deep breathing, accomplished by walking at faster paces for short distances. Also, upper body chest strengthening exercises can help.

✓ Directions of how to do the individual stretches can be found in the Flexibility Chapter.

✓ Directions for how to do the individual strength exercises can be found in the Resistance and Strengthening Chapter.

CHAPTER 16
HEAD AND NECK CANCER

Exercise can improve recovery from head and neck cancer treatments, improve the tolerability of the treatments and lower the risk of developing a new or recurrent head and neck cancer. Head and neck cancers are common cancers that affect the oral and nasal cavities extending all the way down into the larynx, or voice box region of the neck. These do not include the more rare primary brain tumors or thyroid cancers. As previously outlined in this book, exercise improves health and wellbeing in numerous ways which can lower the risk of cancer, including head and neck cancer, and can help both recover from and tolerate the treatments for head and neck cancer including surgery, radiation, and chemotherapy. Whether you have had head and neck cancer and are recovering from or going through treatments, or whether you want to avoid head and neck cancer altogether, exercise should be an important part of your daily routine.

Head and neck cancer treatments can affect people in many ways depending on the treatments received. Some people only require surgery, but others require radiation and/or chemotherapy. There are also people focused on preventing head and neck cancer altogether. This chapter will go into more detail on how exercise can benefit those recovering from treatments for head and neck cancer, going through treatments for head and neck cancer, living with head and neck cancer, or just trying to prevent it altogether. For those who have received treatments for head and neck cancer, there are considerations when exercising that will be outlined in this chapter. At the end of the chapter, I will outline an example work out plan for someone recovering from head and neck cancer treatments.

Exercise plays an important role for people recovering from head and neck cancer treatments, and can likely also prevent occurrences and recurrences of head and neck cancer. Environmental exposures such as alcohol and cigarette smoke are some of the biggest risk factors causing head and neck cancers, so minimizing exposures to these substances are important. Those people who participate in at least 150 minutes of moderate exercise per week are less likely to smoke as much as those who do not exercise. In addition, diabetes has been linked to worse outcomes in people with head and neck cancer undergoing treatments. Exercise has been shown to lower the rates of diabetes and control blood sugar better in those who have diabetes.

Exercise also causes changes in the hormone levels of the body which can improve the tolerability and recovery from treatments for head and neck cancer and lower the risk of occurrence and recurrence of head and neck cancers. Insulin-like growth factor very likely plays an important role in the development of head and neck cancer and is lowered with any type of activity, even stretching which can potentially inhibit cancer cell development. Other hormones including growth hormone, thyroid hormone, epinephrine, insulin and testosterone are involved with strengthening muscles and joints, managing the body's metabolism, and maintaining appropriate weight. Together, these hormones produced during exercise promote wellness of the body and likely all contribute to the lower rates of head and neck cancer and improved tolerability of head and neck cancer treatments. Endorphins are hormones increased in the blood of people who participate in vigorous exercise. Remember that these hormones are structurally similar to morphine and can activate opioid receptors in the brain and elsewhere to minimize pain which may be how they improve arthritis pain and scar tissue pain. In addition, exercise can improve and prevent pain by strengthening the muscles that support the joints putting less stress on those joints. Risks of fractures are reduced by having stronger muscles and healthier joints. Recall also that exercise helps improve coordination and flexibility of the body which can lower the risk of falls. Better body mechanics promote health, lower injuries, and improve and prevent pain. Finally, exercise can improve the sense of well-being by increasing levels of serotonin and norepinephrine during exercise which improves depression and anxiety, and can improve sleep.

For those who have undergone treatment for head and neck cancer, there are certain exercises that are important to improve recovery and long-term wellbeing. Surgery can leave lasting physical changes including scar tissue which can cause tightness of the skin and neck and lead to a stiff and sometimes disfigured neck, called a contracture. Radiation can also lead to similar neck changes. In addition, both surgery and radiation can lead to a dry mouth, difficulty swallowing and taste changes which can lead to weight loss. As you recover from surgery, the surgeon will release you to start increasing your activity usually around 4-6 weeks after surgery. Once you are able to start upper body exercises, start slow and proceed as your body is ready so that you do not cause the surgical incision site to heal more slowly. In addition, radiation may slow your ability to progress with your exercises during the treatments. Stretching your upper body which includes your neck, shoulders, chest, arms and back will be important in your exercise routine and should be done at least 4-5 days per week, and I would suggest daily. Find a time to set aside to do them as part of your daily routine so that you do not forget, such as when you take your shower or just prior to going to bed. Also, remember to use sun screen when you are in the sun for up to 12 months after radiation or chemotherapy as your skin is more sensitive to the sun.

If you are exercising while receiving chemotherapy, then it is important to know the side effects of the specific medicines you are receiving when considering your exercise routine. If the chemotherapy you are receiving can cause fatigue, weakness, or dizziness which all can occur with anemia, then shorten your aerobic exercise that you do at any given time to shorter more frequent intervals at slower paces and make sure to hydrate well prior to, during and after you exercise. Because saliva is often affected by treatments for head and neck cancer, you should get a bottle that is convenient to carry with you while you exercise to drink even during your exercises. If the chemotherapy you are receiving lowers your immune system, then be careful working out with crowds, like at gyms or in large groups. Chemotherapy often leads to bowel changes such as constipation or diarrhea, and sometimes nausea and even vomiting. Staying well hydrated will help with these side effects. Often exercise will actually make these side effects better. Most chemotherapy and radiation will make you more sensitive to the sun for up to a year, so wear sunscreen when you are in the sun for more than about 10 to 15 minutes depending on your skin type. Fair complexions may require sunscreen for even a few minutes of sun exposure. With certain chemotherapies for head and neck cancer, the rashes are improved by wearing sunscreen even while exposed to indoor light. Chemotherapy can cause dry skin and sometimes rashes; excessive sweating can worsen those conditions. Make sure to moisturize your skin and you may need to do short intervals of aerobic exercise to minimize sweating.

When considering all these side effects of head and neck cancer treatments and benefits from exercise, you will want to incorporate the types of exercises into your routine to have a successful exercise program which should include stretching, resistance or strength training, and aerobic endurance exercises. Balance exercises can be incorporated into some of the activities to simplify your routine. Here is an example of an exercise plan for someone recovering from head and neck cancer treatments. This is just an example; certainly modify it to meet your interests, activity level, and access to gyms or equipment.

Example Exercise Plan – Head and Neck Cancer

60 year old man was diagnosed with a posterior tongue head and neck cancer about 12 months ago and had surgery followed by radiation with chemotherapy. He is still struggling with dry mouth and fatigue, but is now also starting to have a stiff neck, shoulder and upper back from tightness of the surgery site in his neck. He still works full time during the week.

Weekly Exercise Plan – beginning

Monday – strength training; stretch upper body and lower body

Tuesday – walk 30 minutes; stretch upper body

Wednesday – strength training; stretch upper body and lower body

Thursday – walk 30 minutes; stretch upper body

Friday – strength training; stretch upper body and lower body

Saturday – bike ride 90 minutes; stretch upper body

Sunday – stretch upper body

Weekly Exercise Plan – after 6 months of increasing walking time

Monday – walk 20 minutes; strength training; stretch upper body and lower body

Tuesday – walk 45 minutes; stretch upper body

Wednesday – walk 20 minutes; strength training; stretch upper body and lower body

Thursday – walk 45 minutes; stretch upper body

Friday – walk 20 minutes; strength training; stretch upper body and lower body

Saturday – walk 45 minutes; stretch upper body

Sunday – walk 45 minutes; stretch upper body

Weekly Reminders:
- ✓ Incorporate daily stretching of his neck and upper body to improve surgical incision pain.
- ✓ Plan to do aerobic exercise at least 4 days per week.
- ✓ Goal of 150 minutes of moderate intensity exercise per week.
- ✓ Incorporate resistance and strengthening at least 3 times per week on non-consecutive days to strengthen muscles and bones and prevent fractures. Since he is under 65 years old, he should plan to do 8-10 different exercises that target all the major muscle groups, performing 8-12 repetitions of each exercise. (If he was over 65 years old, then he should do lighter weights or less resistance and increase the repetitions to 10-15.)

✓ Incorporate flexibility and balance exercises, such as walking on uneven ground, 1 to 2 times per week to help prevent falls.

✓ Wear sunscreen if in the sun for more than 10 minutes since he completed radiation and chemotherapy treatments less than a year ago.

Daily Routine – beginning

Monday, Wednesday and Friday

- walk 20 minutes,
    - goal heart rate 75-127 (50-85% of max heart rate)
- strength training with a resistance band
    - push-ups
    - chest press
    - chest fly
    - pull-aparts
    - standing row
    - forward raise
    - wood choppers
    - trunk rotation
    - bicep curls
    - wall sits
- stretch upper body and lower body
    - neck roll
    - upper shoulder
    - triceps
    - shoulder and chest
    - low back
    - hip flexor and glute

Tuesday, Thursday, Saturday and Sunday

- walk 20 minutes
    - goal heart rate 75-127 (50-85% of max heart rate)
- deep breathing exercises
    - blow up 5-10 standard balloons
- stretch upper body
    - neck roll
    - upper shoulder
    - triceps
    - shoulder and chest

Daily Routine – after 6 months of increasing walking time

Monday, Wednesday and Friday

- walk 20 minutes,
- goal heart rate 75-127 (50-85% of max heart rate)
- strength training with a resistance band
    - push-ups
    - chest press
    - chest fly
    - pull-aparts
    - standing row
    - forward raise
    - wood choppers
    - trunk rotation
    - bicep curls
    - wall sits
- stretch upper body and lower body
    - neck roll
    - upper shoulder
    - triceps

- shoulder and chest
- low back
- hip flexor and glute

Tuesday, Thursday, Saturday and Sunday

- walk 45 minutes total, goal heart rate 75-127 (50-85% of max heart rate), 15 minutes at the lower heart rate goal, then speed up for 5 minutes to get your heart rate at the higher goal level, then 15 minutes at the lower goal, then 5 minutes at the higher goal, then 15 minutes at the lower goal, and then end with 5 minutes at the higher goal.
- stretch upper body
  - neck roll
  - upper shoulder
  - triceps
  - shoulder and chest

Daily Reminders:

- ✓ Warm up and cool down for 2-5 minutes each day around exercises.
- ✓ Hold the stretches for 60 seconds. (If under 65 years old, then for 30 seconds.)
- ✓ Repeat each stretch at least twice and up to 4 times for each side.
- ✓ For strength exercises, chose exercises that will work all the different major muscle groups. Plan a total of 8-10 exercises. Repeat each exercise 2-4 times (sets) for each side. In each set, perform 10-15 repetitions. (If he was under 65 years old, then he should do heavier weights or more resistance and decrease the repetitions to 8-12.)

✓ Maximum heart rate is 220 minus your age. Target heart rate during exercise is your maximum heart rate multiplied by 0.5 and by 0.85 which will give you the target range of 50-85% of your maximum heart rate. Fat burning typically happens at 60-70% maximum heart rate which is your maximum heart rate multiplied by 0.6 and 0.7 to get a range. Weight loss can occur when you reach your fat burning heart rate for at least 15 minutes.

✓ Directions of how to do the stretches can be found in the Flexibility Chapter.

✓ Directions for how to do the strength exercises can be found in the Resistance and Strengthening Chapter.

CHAPTER 17

GYNECOLOGIC CANCER

Exercise can decrease the risk of developing a new or recurrent gynecologic cancer, and improve the tolerability of treatments and recovery from treatments for gynecologic cancer. Gynecologic cancers include the more common cervical, uterine, fallopian tube and ovarian cancers. There are some rarer cancers of the gynecologic system such as vaginal cancer and primary peritoneal cancer which also are included in this section. Some of the lower gynecologic cancers such as cervical and uterine cancers often have radiation and surgery as a major part of their treatment. The other cancers more commonly have surgery and chemotherapy playing a major role in their treatment. Never-the-less, a major modifiable risk factor for most of the gynecologic cancers includes obesity. And as we have discussed previously, exercise can help with weight loss and maintenance of normal weight which can lower the risk of obesity, thereby lowering the risk of gynecologic cancers. In addition, exercise improves health and wellbeing in numerous other ways which can lower the risk of gynecologic cancers, and can help both recover from and tolerate the treatments for gynecologic cancers. Whether you have had a gynecologic cancer and are recovering from or going through treatments, or whether you want to avoid developing a gynecologic cancer altogether, exercise should be an important part of your daily routine.

Many of the gynecologic cancers are in the top ten cancers affecting women. The average age of diagnosis for cervical cancer is in the mid 40's and for uterine and ovarian cancer is in the early 60's, although anyone can develop these cancers. With cervical cancer, surgery and/or radiation is often used for earlier stages of the cancer, although chemotherapy is also sometimes utilized. Uterine cancer also may include surgery, radiation and chemotherapy as important components of the treatment plan. For ovarian, fallopian tube and peritoneal cancers, surgery and chemotherapy are the most common treatments used. Many women want to prevent gynecologic cancers altogether. This chapter will go into more detail on how exercise can specifically prevent gynecologic cancers from developing or recurring, and how it benefits those recovering from treatments for gynecologic cancer, going through treatments for a gynecologic cancer, or living with a gynecologic cancer.

For those who have received treatments for gynecologic cancers, there are considerations when exercising that will be outlined in this chapter. At the end of the chapter, I will outline an example work out plan for someone who has previously received cervical cancer treatments and someone who is receiving ovarian cancer treatments as the symptoms from treatment and exercises can vary slightly.

Gynecologic cancers can be prevented in people who exercise regularly and maintain a normal weight. Research has shown that people who exercise regularly have lower rates of gynecologic cancer occurrences and recurrences. In addition, there are slightly higher rates of uterine cancers in people with diabetes, and exercise has been shown to lower the rates of diabetes and control blood sugar better in those who have diabetes. There is also an association with worse outcomes in people with gynecologic cancers who are obese, and exercise can lower the rates of obesity. When looking at the types of exercise that are beneficial, most types seem to be beneficial, but those focused on maintaining a normal weight seem to offer the most benefit at preventing gynecologic cancers.

One of the risk factors for gynecologic cancers is obesity. Gynecologic cancers such as uterine and ovarian cancers have estrogen receptors on the outside of the cancer cells. When estrogen binds to these receptors, it can stimulate the cancer cells to grow and divide. Estrogen is made in the ovaries and the fatty tissues of the body. The more fatty tissue present, the more estrogen that can be made which thereby can bind to the receptors to stimulate more growth and division of the cancer cells. This is why obesity is linked to higher rates of estrogen driven cancers such as uterine cancer. Exercise can help with weight loss and muscle development to lower levels of body fat which can lower the occurrence and recurrence of estrogen driven cancers such as uterine and ovarian cancer, as well as breast cancer.

There are beneficial hormones that are produced when we exercise and are active. These hormones work in different ways to prevent cancer occurrences and recurrences, and promote well-being. An important hormone lowered when we exercise is insulin-like growth factor which at lower levels can inhibit cancer cell development or growth potentially helping to lower the risk of developing gynecologic cancers, especially ovarian and fallopian tube cancers. Other hormones including growth hormone, thyroid hormone, epinephrine, insulin, and testosterone are involved with managing the body's metabolism, maintaining appropriate weight, promoting lean muscle mass, and strengthening muscles and joints. Together, the hormones produced during exercise promote wellness of the body and likely all contribute to the lower rates of gynecologic cancers and improve recovery from treatments for gynecologic cancers.

Other hormones produced during exercise called endorphins are also increased in the blood of people who participate in moderate to vigorous exercise. Remember that these hormones are structurally similar to morphine and can activate opioid receptors in the brain and elsewhere to minimize pain which may be how they improve arthritis pain and scar tissue pain. In addition, exercise can improve and prevent pain by strengthening the muscles that support the joints putting less stress on those joints. Recall also that exercise helps improve coordination and flexibility of the body which can lower the risk of falls. Better body mechanics promote health, lower injuries, and improve and prevent pain.

People diagnosed with gynecologic cancers and undergoing treatments can develop symptoms that affect well-being in other ways. Exercise can improve the sense of well-being by increasing levels of serotonin and norepinephrine during exercise which improves depression and anxiety, and can improve sleep. If you were diagnosed and treated for a gynecologic cancer when you were premenopausal, then the treatments may induce earlier than anticipated menopause which can lead to menopausal symptoms such as hot flashes, irritability and weaker bones at a younger age than anticipated. Incorporating some strengthening, flexibility and balance exercises will help keep the bones strong and prevent falls and fractures. Exercise can actually improve menopausal symptoms. Weight gain is common after surgery and chemotherapy which can be countered by regular aerobic exercise focusing on keeping your target heart rate range in the 60% to 70% of your maximum heart rate range for at least 15 minutes per session which is where fat burning occurs.

For those who have undergone treatment for a gynecologic cancer, there are certain exercises that can help to improve recovery and long-term wellbeing. Surgery can leave lasting physical changes including scar tissue, chronic pain and urinary incontinence. Radiation given to the pelvis can sometimes cause chronic loose stools or even diarrhea and can sometimes make scar tissue worse. Dehydration can occur easily if you have chronic diarrhea so staying well hydrated is very important. In addition, both surgery and radiation can lead to chronic swelling in the legs called lymphedema. You should avoid abdominal or pelvic floor exercises until you have healed enough from surgery. Since different surgeries can have different recovery rates, check with your surgeon as to when you could start an exercise program that might cause jarring or stress to the abdomen and pelvis. Once you start the abdomen and lower body exercises, start slowly and proceed as your body is ready so that you do not delay healing. You may need to get an abdominal binder or at least wear a tight undergarment during exercises that prevent hernias from developing after abdominal surgeries. However, abdominal and pelvic floor exercises are very important to controlling pain from scar tissue, improving urinary continence, preventing swelling in your legs, and providing long term good quality of life, so these are important exercises to have in your daily routine.

If you are exercising while receiving chemotherapy, then it is important to know the side effects of the specific medicines you are receiving when considering your exercise routine. If the chemotherapy you are receiving can cause fatigue, weakness, or dizziness which can also occur with anemia, then shorten your aerobic exercise that you do at any given time to shorter more frequent intervals at slower paces and make sure to hydrate well prior to, during and after you exercise. In this situation, you may also need to do less weight or resistance when doing strengthening exercises. You can still stay toned by doing more repetitions of lighter weights during this time. If the chemotherapy you are receiving lowers your immune system, then be careful working out with crowds, like at gyms or in large groups. Not only does surgery and radiation for gynecologic cancers lead to bowel changes like constipation and diarrhea, but chemotherapy can compound these symptoms or change the symptoms. Staying well hydrated will help with these side effects. However, nausea, vomiting, and heartburn can occur which can affect your ability to stay well hydrated. During these situations, hydrating with electrolyte fluids may help more than water if you plan to do aerobic exercises. There are some types of chemotherapy given for gynecologic cancers that can cause numbness and tingling in the hands or feet. Being careful with balance exercises during this time is important, but exercise can actually often improve these symptoms as well. If you are receiving a type of chemotherapy sometimes used for gynecologic cancers that can increase the risk of bleeding, then avoid activities that might increase your risk of falling. Most chemotherapy will make you more sensitive to the sun for at least 6 months and up to a year after completing the chemotherapy, so wear sunscreen when you are in the sun for more than about 10 to 15 minutes depending on your skin type. Fair complexions may require sunscreen for even a few minutes of sun exposure. Chemotherapy can cause dry skin and sometimes rashes; excessive sweating can worsen those conditions. Make sure to moisturize your skin and you may need to do shorter intervals of aerobic exercise to minimize sweating until you have recovered from the chemotherapy side effects.

Once you understand all the potential side effects of treatment for gynecologic cancers and the benefits of exercise, planning the types of exercises to incorporate into your routine helps you come up with a successful program which should include aerobic endurance exercises, resistance or strength training and stretching. Balance exercises can be incorporated into some of the activities to simplify your routine. The aerobic exercises should be aimed at attaining and maintaining a normal weight. So what might an exercise plan look like for someone who has received treatment for cervical cancer or is undergoing treatment for ovarian cancer? Here are some examples to consider, but certainly modify it to meet your interests, activity level, and access to gyms or equipment.

Example Exercise Plan – Cervical Cancer

40 year old female with cervical cancer treated with surgery now 1 year out from treatment with severe hot flashes, fatigue and weight gain of 25 pounds. She has 2 kids ages 12 and 14 who are busy in school, with sports, and she works full time 40 hours per week.

Weekly Exercise Plan – during the kids' school year

Monday – walk 45 minutes in the park where her child has practice; stretch lower body

Tuesday –strength training; stretch lower/upper body

Wednesday – walk 45 minutes in the park where her child has practice; stretch lower body

Thursday –strength training; stretch lower/upper body

Friday – walk 20 minutes at lunch during break at work; stretch lower body

Saturday – walk 45 minutes; stretch lower/upper body

Sunday – walk 45 minutes; stretch lower body

Weekly Exercise Plan – during summer

Monday – bike to work and home 40 minutes; stretch lower body

Tuesday –bike to work and home 40 minutes; strength training; stretch lower/upper body

Wednesday – bike to work and home 40 minutes; stretch lower body

Thursday –bike to work and home 40 minutes; strength training; stretch lower/upper body

Friday – bike to work and home 40 minutes; stretch lower body

Saturday – walk in park 45 minutes; stretch lower body

Sunday – swim in afternoon 30 minutes; stretch lower/upper body

Weekly Reminders:
- ✓ Incorporate abdominal and pelvic floor stretching at least 5 times per week but preferably daily to maintain good urinary control.
- ✓ Plan to do aerobic exercise 5 days per week to lose weight and then maintain normal weight. Goal heart rate is 60-70% of maximum heart rate for at least 15 minutes to help burn fat and maintain a normal weight.
- ✓ Goal of 150 minutes of moderate intensity exercise per week.
- ✓ Incorporate resistance and strengthening at least 3 times per week on non-consecutive days to strengthen muscles and bones and prevent fractures. Since she is under 65 years old, she should plan to do 8-10 different exercises that target all the major muscle groups, performing 8-12 repetitions of each

exercise. (If she was over 65 years old, then she should do lighter weights or less resistance and increase the repetitions to 10-15.)

✓ Incorporate flexibility and balance exercises, such as walking on uneven ground, 1 to 2 times per week to help prevent falls.

Daily Routine – during school year

Monday, Wednesday and Sunday

- walk 45 minutes in the park where her child has practice,
  - goal heart rate of 108-126 (60-70% max heart rate)
- stretch lower body
  - hip flexor/quadriceps/back/calf combined stretch
  - low back/abdomen stretch

Tuesday and Thursday

- strength training
  - high plank
  - side plank body rotations
  - squats
  - lunges
  - bicep curls with a band
  - triceps kickbacks with a band
  - twists
  - leg lifts
- stretch lower body and upper body
  - hip flexor/quadriceps/back/calf combined stretch
  - low back/abdomen stretch
  - triceps
  - shoulder and chest

Friday

- walk 20 minutes at lunch during break at work,
  - goal heart rate of 108-126 (60-70% max heart rate)
- stretch lower body
  - hip flexor/quadriceps/back/calf combined stretch
  - low back/abdomen stretch

Saturday

- walk 45 minutes,
  - goal heart rate of 108-126 (60-70% max heart rate)
- strength training
  - high plank
  - side plank body rotations
  - squats
  - lunges
  - bicep curls with a band
  - triceps kickbacks with a band
  - twists
  - leg lifts
- stretch lower body and upper body
  - hip flexor/quadriceps/back/calf combined stretch
  - low back/abdomen stretch
  - triceps
  - shoulders and chest

Sunday

- walk 45 minutes,
  - goal heart rate of 108-126 (60-70% max heart rate)
- stretch lower body
  - hip flexor/quadriceps/back/calf combined stretch
  - low back/abdomen stretch

Daily Routine – during summer

Monday, Wednesday and Friday

- bike to work, 20 minutes, goal heart rate of 108-126 (60-70% max heart rate)
- bike home, 20 minutes, goal heart rate of 108-126 (60-70% max heart rate)
- stretch lower body after ride home
    - hip flexor/quadriceps/back/calf combined stretch
    - low back/abdomen stretch

Tuesday and Thursday

- bike to work, 20 minutes, goal heart rate of 108-126 (60-70% max heart rate)
- bike home, 20 minutes, goal heart rate of 108-126 (60-70% max heart rate)
- strength training upper body
    - high plank
    - plank shoulder taps
    - side plank body rotations
    - bicep curls with a band
    - triceps kickback with a band
    - twists
- stretch lower body and upper body after ride home
    - hip flexor/quadriceps/back/calf combined stretch
    - low back/abdomen stretch
    - triceps
    - shoulder and chest

Saturday

- walk in park 45 minutes, goal heart rate of 108-126 (60-70% max heart rate)
- stretch lower body
  - hip flexor/quadriceps/back/calf combined stretch
  - low back/abdomen stretch

Sunday

- swim in afternoon 30 minutes, goal heart rate of 108-126 (60-70% max heart rate)
- stretch lower and upper body
  - hip flexor/quadriceps/back/calf combined stretch
  - low back/abdomen stretch
  - triceps
  - shoulders and chest

Daily Reminders:

- ✓ Warm up and cool down for 2-5 minutes each day around exercises.
- ✓ Hold the stretches for 30 seconds. (If over 65 years old, then hold the stretch for 60 seconds.)
- ✓ Repeat each stretch at least twice and up to 4 times for each side.
- ✓ For resistance exercises, chose strengthening exercises that will work all the different major muscle groups. Plan at least 8-10 different exercises. Repeat each exercise 2-4 times (sets) for each side. In each set, perform 8-12 repetitions. (If over 65 years old, then perform 10-15 reps using lighter weights.)
- ✓ Maximum heart rate is 220 minus your age. Target heart rate during exercise is your maximum heart rate multiplied by 0.5 and by 0.85 which will give you the target range of 50-85% of your

maximum heart rate. Fat burning typically happens at 60-70% maximum heart rate which is your maximum heart rate multiplied by 0.6 and 0.7 to get a range. Weight loss can occur when you reach your fat burning heart rate for at least 15 minutes.

✓ Biking fulfills leg strength training. Swimming fulfills core and upper body strength training.

✓ Directions of how to do the individual stretches can be found in the Flexibility Chapter.

✓ Directions for how to do the individual strength exercises can be found in the Resistance and Strengthening Chapter.

CHAPTER 18

BLADDER AND KIDNEY CANCER

Exercise can improve recovery from bladder and kidney cancer treatments, improve the tolerability of the treatments and lower the risk of developing a new or recurrent bladder and kidney cancer. Some kidney cancers are very similar to bladder cancers, but others are quite different. This can lead to different medicines used to treat this cancer, but the surgery, when indicated is similar. As previously outlined in this book, exercise improves health and wellbeing in numerous ways which can lower the risk of cancer, including bladder and kidney cancers, and can help both recover from and tolerate the treatments for bladder and kidney cancers such as surgery, radiation, and chemotherapy. Whether you have had a bladder or kidney cancer and are recovering from or going through treatments, or whether you want to avoid developing a bladder or kidney cancer altogether, exercise should be an important part of your daily routine.

Bladder cancer tends to be more common than kidney cancer. They are in the top ten cancers affecting both women and men. The average age of diagnosis is between 60-70 years old for most bladder and kidney cancers. Surgery is very often the primary treatment for both bladder and kidney cancers, and when they are caught early enough may be the only treatment needed. With kidney cancer, surgery is usually one of the first treatments, but for bladder cancer, surgery may occur before or after treatments with chemotherapy. Radiation is occasionally needed for bladder cancer, but not commonly used in kidney cancer treatment. There are also many people trying to avoid an early stage bladder cancer from progressing or trying to prevent bladder and kidney cancer altogether.

This chapter will go into more detail on how exercise can specifically prevent bladder and kidney cancers, and how it benefits those people recovering from treatments for both bladder and kidney cancer, those going through treatments for a bladder or kidney cancer, or those living with bladder or kidney cancer. For those people who have received treatments for bladder or kidney cancers, there are considerations when exercising that will be outlined in this chapter. At the end of the chapter, I will outline an example work out plan for someone who has previously received bladder cancer treatments and someone who has received kidney cancer treatments as the symptoms from treatment and exercises can vary slightly.

As has been previously discussed, there are a lot of hormones that are produced when we exercise and are active. These hormones work in different ways to prevent cancer occurrences and recurrences. When considering bladder and kidney cancers, insulin-like growth factor is likely one of the more important hormones lowered during all types of activities potentially inhibiting cancer cell growth and development. Other hormones including growth hormone, thyroid hormone, epinephrine, insulin, and testosterone are involved with managing the body's metabolism, maintaining appropriate weight, and strengthening muscles and joints. Together, the hormones produced during exercise promote wellness of the body and likely all contribute to the lower rates of bladder and kidney cancers, and importantly, improve tolerance of cancer treatments and recovery after treatments.

Other hormones that are produced during exercise called endorphins are also increased in the blood of people who participate in moderate to vigorous exercise. Remember that these hormones are structurally similar to morphine and can activate opioid receptors in the brain and elsewhere to minimize pain which may be how they improve scar tissue pain which can commonly occur after surgery for bladder and kidney cancer. In addition, exercise can improve and prevent pain by strengthening the muscles that support the joints putting less stress on those joints, including the large joints in the pelvis. Recall also that exercise helps improve coordination and flexibility of the body which can lower the risk of falls. Better body mechanics promote health, lower injuries, and improve and prevent pain.

So keeping all this in consideration when thinking about types of exercises to incorporate into your routine helps come up with a successful program which should include aerobic endurance exercises, resistance or strength training, and stretching. Balance exercises can be incorporated into some of the activities to simplify your routine. There are other considerations when developing your exercise routine based on treatments that may have been required for your bladder or kidney cancer.

For those who have undergone treatment for a bladder or kidney cancer, there are certain exercises that can help you to recover and maintain wellbeing. Surgery can leave lasting physical changes including scar tissue, ostomy bags, and sometimes chronic pain. Radiation given to the abdomen or pelvis can sometimes cause chronic urinary incontinence, loose stools or even diarrhea, and can sometimes make scar tissue worse. Dehydration can occur easily if you have chronic diarrhea. You should avoid abdominal or pelvic floor exercises until you have healed enough from surgery. Since different surgeries can have different recovery rates, check with your surgeon as to when you could start an exercise program that might cause jarring or stress to the abdomen and pelvis. Once you start the abdomen and lower body exercises, start slowly and proceed as your body is ready so that you do not delay healing. You may need to get an abdominal binder or at least wear a tight undergarment during exercises that prevent hernias from developing after abdominal surgeries. If you have an ostomy bag, consider doing abdominal exercises that are strengthening your back muscles more than exercises that are focused on the front abdominal muscles to avoid hernias. However, abdominal and pelvic floor exercises are very important to controlling pain from scar tissue and providing long term good quality of life, so these are important exercises to have in your daily routine.

If you are exercising while receiving chemotherapy, then it is important to know the side effects of the specific medicines you are receiving when considering your exercise routine. If the chemotherapy you are receiving can cause fatigue, weakness, or dizziness which can also occur with anemia, then shorten your aerobic exercise that you do at any given time to shorter more frequent intervals at slower paces and make sure to hydrate well prior to, during and after you exercise. In this situation, you may also need to do less weight or resistance when doing strengthening exercises. You can still stay toned by doing more repetitions of lighter weights during this time. If the chemotherapy you are receiving lowers your immune system, then be careful working out with crowds, like at gyms or in large groups. Not only can surgery and radiation for bladder and kidney cancers lead to urinary changes, but chemotherapy can lead to bowel changes such as constipation or diarrhea which can compound symptoms you are dealing with as you exercise. Sometimes, nausea or vomiting can occur, or the liquids and foods that you take in have to be modified due to side effects from the treatments. Staying well hydrated will help with these side effects. Try to hydrate just before, during and after exercising, but avoid eating within about 45 to 60 minutes prior to and after exercising to help with these symptoms during your exercise routine. Often exercise will actually make these side effects better. If you have dizziness, be careful with balance exercises, but balance exercises can still be beneficial. Most chemotherapy will make you more sensitive to the sun for at least 6 months and up to a year, so wear sunscreen when you are in the sun for more than about 10 to 15 minutes depending on your skin type. Fair complexions may require sunscreen for even a few minutes of sun exposure. Chemotherapy can cause dry skin and sometimes rashes; excessive sweating can worsen those conditions. Make sure to moisturize your skin and you may need to do short intervals of aerobic exercise to minimize sweating.

People diagnosed with bladder and kidney cancers and undergoing treatments can develop symptoms that affect well-being in other ways. Exercise can improve the sense of well-being by increasing levels of serotonin and norepinephrine during exercise which improves depression and anxiety, and can improve sleep. Incorporating some strengthening, flexibility and balance exercises will help keep the bones strong and prevent falls and fractures. Often weight loss is a problem after bladder and kidney surgery. Try to focus on strengthening and lower intensity workouts to prevent too much weight loss.

So what might an exercise plan look like for someone who is undergoing treatment for bladder cancer or has received treatment for kidney cancer? Here are some examples to consider, but certainly modify it to meet your interests, activity level, and access to gyms or equipment.

Example Exercise Plan – Bladder Cancer

65 year old man with bladder cancer treated with surgery, cystectomy, is now undergoing chemotherapy. They were unable to build him an artificial bladder and so he has a urostomy bag. He is struggling with weight gain from lack of activity and nausea which still lingers from surgery and due to chemotherapy. He has fatigue from his chemotherapy.

Weekly Exercise Plan – beginning

Monday – walk 10 minutes in the morning and 10 minutes in the evening; stretch lower body

Tuesday –strength training; stretch lower body and upper body

Wednesday – walk 10 minutes in the morning and 10 minutes in the evening; stretch lower body

Thursday – strength training; stretch lower body and upper body

Friday – walk 10 minutes in the morning and 10 minutes in the evening; stretch lower body

Saturday – strength training; stretch lower body and upper body

Sunday –stretch lower body

Weekly Exercise Plan – as stamina increases

Monday – walk 20-30 minutes; stretch lower body

Tuesday –strength training; stretch lower body and upper body

Wednesday – walk 20-30 minutes; stretch lower body

Thursday –strength training; stretch lower body and upper body

Friday – walk 20-30 minutes; stretch lower body

Saturday – strength training; stretch lower body and upper body

Sunday – walk 10-30 minutes; stretch lower body

Weekly Reminders:

✓ Incorporate abdominal and pelvic floor stretching at least 5 times per week but preferably daily to maintain good bowel function, and if he had been able to have an artificial bladder built, to help with urinary function and control.

✓ Abdominal exercises will focus more on back strengthening since he has a urostomy bag, but this is true even if he had an artificial bladder.

✓ Plan to do aerobic exercise 3 days per week for cardiovascular health but minimize weight loss. Goal heart rate is 50% of maximum heart rate for at least 15 minutes. The lower heart rate goal is to avoid dehydration and too much weight loss, but still get the other health benefits from aerobic exercise.

✓ Goal of 60 minutes of light intensity exercise per week right now while on chemotherapy. Eventually, the goal will increase to 150 minutes of moderate intensity exercise per week.

✓ Incorporate resistance and strengthening at least 3 times per week on non-consecutive days to strengthen muscles and bones and prevent fractures. Since he is 65 years old, he should plan to do 8-10 different exercises that target all the major muscle groups, performing 10-15 repetitions of each exercise. (If he was under 65 years old, then he should do heavier weights or more resistance and lower the repetitions to 8-12.)

✓ Incorporate flexibility and balance exercises 1 to 2 times per week to help prevent falls.

Daily Routine – beginning

Monday, Wednesday, Friday and Sunday

- walk 10 minutes, goal heart rate of 78 (50% max heart rate)
- stretch lower body
  - low back stretch
  - hip flexor and glute stretch
  - adductor leg stretch
  - hamstring stretch
  - quadriceps stretch
  - calf stretch

Tuesday, Thursday and Saturday

- strength training (10-15 reps in 2-4 sets of each) using resistance bands at home
  - biceps curls
  - triceps kickback
  - trunk rotations
  - side bend
  - calf raises
  - wall plank (using body weight for resistance)
  - arm circles (without bands)
- stretch lower body
  - low back stretch
  - hip flexor and glute stretch
  - adductor leg stretch
  - hamstring stretch
  - quadriceps stretch
  - calf stretch

- stretch upper body
    - neck roll
    - upper shoulder stretch
    - triceps stretch
    - shoulder and chest stretch

Daily Routine – advance the training by increasing the length of time walking and types of exercises

Monday, Wednesday, Friday and Sunday

- walk 20 minutes, goal heart rate of 78 (50% max heart rate)
- stretch lower body
    - low back stretch
    - hip flexor and glute stretch
    - adductor leg stretch
    - hamstring stretch
    - quadriceps stretch
    - calf stretch

Tuesday, Thursday and Saturday

- strength training (10-15 reps in 2-4 sets of each) using resistance bands at home
    - biceps curls
    - triceps kickbacks
    - overhead press
    - trunk rotations
    - side bend
    - twists
    - chest fly
    - wall sits without a band
    - forward lunges without a band

- ○ calf raises
- stretch lower body
  - ○ low back stretch
  - ○ hip flexor and glute stretch
  - ○ adductor leg stretch
  - ○ hamstring stretch
  - ○ quadriceps stretch
  - ○ calf stretch
- stretch upper body
  - ○ neck roll
  - ○ upper shoulder stretch
  - ○ triceps stretch
  - ○ shoulder and chest stretch

Daily Reminders:

✓ Warm up and cool down for 2-5 minutes each day around exercises.

✓ Hold the stretches for 60 seconds. (If under 65 years old, then hold the stretch for 30 seconds.)

✓ Repeat each stretch at least twice and up to 4 times for each side.

✓ For resistance exercises, chose strengthening exercises that will work all the different major muscle groups. Plan at least 8-10 different exercises. Repeat each exercise 2-4 times (sets) for each side. In each set, perform 10-15 repetitions. (If under 65 years old, perform 8-12 reps with heavier weights.)

✓ Maximum heart rate is 220 minus your age. Target heart rate during exercise is your maximum heart rate multiplied by 0.5 and by 0.85 which will give you the target range of 50-85% of your maximum heart rate. Fat burning typically happens at 60-70% maximum heart rate which is your maximum heart rate multiplied by 0.6 and 0.7 to get a range. Weight loss can occur when you reach your fat burning heart rate for at least 15 minutes.

✓ Directions of how to do the individual stretches can be found in the Flexibility Chapter.

✓ Directions for how to do the individual strength exercises can be found in the Resistance and Strengthening Chapter.

Example Exercise Plan – Kidney Cancer

57 year old woman with kidney cancer treated with surgery 2 months ago. She did not require any other treatment after her surgery. She has had clearance to exercise but she has never regularly exercised in the past.

Weekly Exercise Plan – increase walking time as stamina increases

Monday – walk 15 minutes; lower body strength training; stretch lower body

Tuesday –walk 15 minutes; upper body strength training; stretch lower and upper body

Wednesday – walk 15 minutes; lower body strengthening; stretch lower body

Thursday –walk 15 minutes; upper body strength training; stretch lower and upper body

Friday – walk 15 minutes; lower body strengthening; stretch lower body

Saturday – walk 15 minutes; upper body strength training; stretch lower and upper body

Sunday – walk 15 minutes; stretch lower body

Weekly Reminders:

✓ Incorporate abdominal stretching at least 5 times per week but preferably daily.

✓ Plan to do daily aerobic exercise daily. If she is overweight, then she should have a goal heart rate of 60-70% of her maximum heart rate for at least 15 minutes to help burn fat and maintain a normal weight. If she is not overweight, then she should have a goal heart rate of 50-85% of her maximum heart rate.

✓ Goal of 150 minutes of aerobic exercise per week but since she has not regularly exercised and is likely deconditioned from surgery, she should start with a goal of 90 minutes and work up to a goal of 150 minutes per week.

✓ Incorporate resistance and strengthening at least 3 times per week on non-consecutive days to strengthen muscles and bones and prevent fractures. Since she is under 65 years old, she should plan to do 8-10 different exercises that target all the major muscle groups, performing 8-12 repetitions of each exercise. (If she was over 65 years old, then she should do lighter weights or less resistance and increase the repetitions to 10-15.) She will need to start with low amount of weight or resistance since she has not regularly done exercise.

✓ Incorporate flexibility and balance exercises, such as walking on uneven ground, 1 to 2 times per week to help prevent falls.

✓ She now only has one kidney so avoiding dehydration is very important. She should try to drink 16 ounces of water an hour to two hours before any exercise, and then 8 ounces prior to exercise and about every 15 minutes during the exercise routine and again after exercise.

Daily Routine

Monday, Wednesday and Friday

- walk the amount of time per week goal, goal heart rate 82-134 (50-85% maximum heart rate)
- strength training lower body (just body weight as resistance to start)
  - wall sits
  - lunges
  - calf raises
- stretch lower body
  - hamstring stretch
  - quadriceps stretch
  - adductor leg stretch
  - hip flexor and glute stretch
  - low back stretch

Tuesday, Thursday and Saturday

- walk the amount of time per week goal, goal heart rate 82-134 (50-85% maximum heart rate)
- strength training upper body
  - plank
  - flying
  - arm circles
  - bicep curls with resistance band
  - triceps kickbacks with resistance band
- stretch upper body
  - neck roll
  - upper shoulder stretch
  - triceps stretch
  - shoulder and chest stretch

- stretch lower body
  - hamstring stretch
  - quadriceps stretch
  - adductor leg stretch
  - hip flexor and glute stretch
  - low back stretch

Sunday

- walk the amount of time per week goal, goal heart rate 82-134 (50-85% maximum heart rate)
  - stretch lower body
  - hamstring stretch
  - quadriceps stretch
  - adductor leg stretch
  - hip flexor and glute stretch
  - low back stretch

Daily Reminders:

- ✓ Warm up and cool down for 2-5 minutes each day around exercises.
- ✓ Hold the stretches for 30 seconds. (If over 65 years old, then hold the stretch for 60 seconds.)
- ✓ Repeat each stretch at least twice and up to 4 times for each side.
- ✓ For resistance exercises, choose strengthening exercises that will work all the different major muscle groups. Plan at least 8-10 exercises. Repeat each exercise 2-4 times (sets) for each side. In each set, perform 8-12 repetitions. She will need to start with low resistance or less weight since she has not regularly exercised. (If over 65 years old, then perform 10-15 reps with lighter weights.)
- ✓ She now only has one kidney so avoiding dehydration is very important. She should try to drink 16 ounces of water an hour

to two hours before any exercise, and then 8 ounces prior to exercise and about every 15 minutes during the exercise routine and again after exercise.

✓ Maximum heart rate is 220 minus your age. Target heart rate during exercise is your maximum heart rate multiplied by 0.5 and by 0.85 which will give you the target range of 50-85% of your maximum heart rate. Fat burning typically happens at 60-70% maximum heart rate which is your maximum heart rate multiplied by 0.6 and 0.7 to get a range. Weight loss can occur when you reach your fat burning heart rate for at least 15 minutes.

✓ Directions of how to do the individual stretches can be found in the Flexibility Chapter.

✓ Directions for how to do the individual strength exercises can be found in the Resistance and Strengthening Chapter.

CHAPTER 19

BLOOD CANCERS
AND LYMPHOMAS

Exercise can improve the tolerability and recovery from blood cancer and lymphoma treatments. Exercise can also sometimes lower the risk of developing blood cancers and lymphomas or lower the risk of recurrence or progression of them. Blood cancers include acute leukemias, chronic leukemias, and myeloproliferative disorders like myelodysplasia. In this section, leukemia will be considered interchangeable with blood cancer even though there are a lot of different names given to cancers of the blood and bone marrow. Lymphomas include aggressive lymphomas like diffuse large B cell lymphoma and more slow growing, indolent lymphomas like follicular lymphoma. Some chronic leukemias and indolent lymphomas are significantly influenced by the immune system, such that a healthy immune system can help to control these conditions. Exercise plays an important role in keeping the immune system healthy. Since there are hundreds of different types of blood cancers and lymphomas, it is beyond the scope of this book to discuss each individually in detail. However, this chapter will provide a general guideline of how to approach exercise in the setting of blood cancers and lymphomas depending on the overall condition and type of treatment, if any, being used. For those who are receiving or recently received treatments for leukemia or lymphoma, there are considerations when exercising that will be outlined in this chapter as well. At the end of the chapter, I will provide an example work out plan for someone who has previously received intensive treatments for a leukemia or lymphoma and for someone who is on a less intensive chemotherapy which is ongoing. Exercise alone is unlikely to prevent the need for treatment, but when used with other healthy lifestyle choices, it may delay the time that treatment is needed for some forms of blood cancers, or leukemias, and lymphoma.

As previously outlined in this book, exercise improves health and wellbeing in numerous ways which can lower the risk of cancer, including some types of low grade leukemias and lymphomas. In addition, exercise can help both recover from and tolerate the treatments for leukemia and lymphoma. Most of the treatments for blood cancers and lymphomas are forms of chemotherapy and immunotherapy with a lot of different side effects which may be able to be improved with exercise. Whether you have a leukemia or lymphoma, are recovering from or going through treatments for one of them, or whether you are trying to avoid developing a leukemia or lymphoma altogether, exercise should be an important part of your daily routine.

When we exercise, there are a lot of hormones that are produced that work in different ways to prevent cancer occurrences and recurrences. When considering cancers of the blood and bone marrow and lymphomas, the different hormones produced during exercise can assist the body to lower the rates of developing some types of leukemias and lymphomas, and improve recovery from the treatments for these cancers. These hormones which include insulin-like growth factor, growth hormone, thyroid hormone, epinephrine, insulin, and testosterone are involved with managing the body's metabolism, maintaining appropriate weight, and strengthening muscles and joints. Together, the hormones produced during exercise promote wellness of the body and likely all contribute to lowering the rates of leukemia and lymphoma, and importantly, improving toler-ance of cancer treatments and recovery after treatments.

Other hormones that are produced during exercise called endorphins are increased in the blood of people who participate in moderate to vigorous exercise. Remember that these hormones are structurally similar to morphine and can activate opioid receptors in the brain and elsewhere to minimize pain and improve mood and depression. In addition, exercise can strengthen the muscles that support the joints leading to less stress on those joints, including the large joints in the pelvis. Since generalized weakness is common when receiv-ing treatments for leukemias and lymphomas, this can help to lower the risk of injuries. Recall also that exercise helps improve coordina-tion and flexibility of the body which can lower the risk of falls. Better body mechanics promote health, lower the possibility of injuries, and improve and prevent pain.

When considering all these hormonal and other benefits of exercise on wellness, which also can support the immune system, it can help determine the types of exercises to incorporate into your routine to come up with a successful program which should include aerobic exercises, resistance or strength training, and stretching. Balance exercises can be incorporated into some of the activities to simplify your routine.

For those who are undergoing treatment for a blood cancer or lym-phoma with chemotherapy or immunotherapy, it is important to know the side effects of the specific medicines you are receiving when considering your exercise routine. There are a lot of various side effects that could be experienced by all the different medicines. This is a guideline to help with the most common of these side effects during exercise. If the chemotherapy you are receiving can cause fatigue, weakness, or dizziness which can also occur with anemia from the cancer itself, then shorten your aerobic exercise that you do at any given time to shorter more frequent intervals at slower paces and make sure to hydrate well prior to, during and after you exercise. In this situation, you may also need to do less weight or resistance when doing strengthening exercises. You can still stay toned by doing more repetitions of lighter weights during this time. Rarely, the treatments can cause heart dysfunction or irregular rhythm which can lead to symptoms such as increased shortness of breath, swelling in the legs, racing heart, or even chest pain. If the chest pain or racing heart symptoms happen during exercise, then stop exercising immediately and if it does not quickly go away, call emergency support services or go to the hospital to be evaluated. If the symptoms go away, or you have other concerning symptoms that may be related to your heart function, then contact your healthcare provider to be evaluated before continuing with any exercise program. If the chemotherapy you are receiving lowers your immune system, then be careful working out with crowds, like at gyms or in large groups. Chemotherapy can cause bowel changes such as constipation or diarrhea which can sometimes require you to limit or change your exercises to accommodate those symptoms, or at least be near a restroom. If you have nausea or vomiting, then avoid lots of head movement during exercise and stay well hydrated. Try to hydrate just before, during and after exercising, and avoid eating within about 45 to 60 minutes prior to and after exercising to help with nausea and vomiting symptoms. Often exercise will actually make these side effects better. If you have dizziness, be careful with balance exercises, but balance exercises can still be beneficial. Most chemotherapy will make you more sensitive to the sun for at least 6 months and up to a year, so wear sunscreen when you are in the sun for more than about 10 to 15 minutes depending on your skin type. Fair complexions may require sunscreen for even a few minutes of sun exposure. Hats and long sleeved shirts and long pants can help protect the skin as well. Chemotherapy can cause dry skin and sometimes rashes. Excessive sweating or chlorinated pools can worsen those skin conditions. Make sure to moisturize your skin and you may need to do short intervals of aerobic exercise to minimize sweating. Rinse off immediately after exiting a chlorinated pool. Some of the types of chemotherapy and treatments require a central venous catheter that cannot get wet. This may limit your ability to submerge in water and swim. Check with your healthcare providers if you have one of these blood catheters.

People diagnosed with blood cancers and lymphomas undergoing treatments can have symptoms that affect well-being in other ways that exercise can benefit. While exercising, levels of serotonin and norepinephrine increase which can improve depression and anxiety, and can improve sleep. Incorporating some strengthening, flexibility and balance exercises will help keep the bones strong and prevent falls and fractures and improve independence during daily living activities. Often weight loss is a problem with blood cancers and lymphomas. Exercise can improve appetite although avoiding excessive aerobic exercise may be necessary to prevent more weight loss. Focusing on strengthening and lower intensity workouts can promote muscle building, and these exercises also stimulate beneficial hormone productions.

So what might an exercise plan look like for someone who is undergoing treatment for leukemia or has received treatment for lymphoma? Here are some examples to consider, but certainly modify it to meet your interests, activity level, and access to gyms or equipment.

Example Exercise Plan – Hodgkin's Lymphoma

26 year old woman with Hodgkin's lymphoma is treated with chemo-therapy for 4 months followed by radiation therapy to the neck and chest and has just completed the radiation 3 months ago. She is still having problems with hair loss, fatigue, anemia, and a poor appetite.

Weekly Exercise Plan – increase walking time each week as stamina increases

Monday – walk 15 minutes; stretch upper body

Tuesday – walk 15 minutes; balance and resistance training; stretch upper/lower body

Wednesday – walk 15 minutes; stretch upper body

Thursday – walk 15 minutes; balance and resistance training; stretch upper/lower body

Friday – walk 15 minutes; stretch upper body

Saturday – walk 20 minutes with her friend; stretch upper body

Sunday – walk 15 minutes; balance and resistance training; stretch upper/lower body

Weekly Reminders:
- ✓ Incorporate daily stretching of her upper body at a minimum to help recover from the radiation side effects. Lower body stretching should be done at least 3 times weekly.
- ✓ Plan to do daily aerobic exercise to improve her energy and mood. Goal heart rate is 50-85% of maximum heart rate for at least 15 minutes per day. Since she still has anemia, starting at

a slower pace and working to a more advanced pace would be best.

✓ Goal of 150 minutes of moderate intensity exercise per week once her anemia is better.

✓ Incorporate resistance and strengthening at least 3 times per week on non-consecutive days to strengthen muscles and bones and prevent fractures. Since she is under 65 years old, she should plan to do 8-10 different exercises that target all the major muscle groups, performing 8-12 repetitions of each exercise. (If she was over 65 years old, then she should do lighter weights or less resistance and increase the repetitions to 10-15.)

✓ Incorporate flexibility and balance exercises 1 to 2 times per week to help prevent falls.

✓ Wear sunscreen if in the sun for more than 10 minutes since she completed chemotherapy and radiation treatments less than a year ago.

✓ Hydrate well prior to, during and after exercise since radiation and chemotherapy effects which contribute to dehydration can persist for up to 6 months.

Daily Routine

Monday, Wednesday, Friday and Saturday

- walk number of minutes based on weekly plan with a goal heart rate of 97-116 (50-60%)
    - maximum target heart rate to avoid more weight loss)
- stretch upper body
    - neck roll
    - upper shoulder stretch
    - triceps stretch
    - shoulder and chest stretch

Tuesday, Thursday and Sunday
- walk number of minutes based on weekly plan with a goal heart rate of 97-116 (50-60%
- maximum target heart rate to avoid more weight loss)
    - resistance training using body weight exercises except biceps (8-12 reps; 2-4 sets of each)
    - low plank
    - swimmers
    - flying
    - arm circles
    - biceps using 5 pound free weights
    - triceps dips
    - reverse crunches
    - hip raises
    - wall sits
    - lunges (also covers balance)
- stretch upper body
    - neck roll
    - upper shoulder stretch
    - triceps stretch
    - shoulder and chest stretch
- stretch lower body
    - low back/hips/hamstrings/glutes
    - hip flexors/quadriceps/back/calf (also covers balance)

Advance
- When feeling ready to change aerobic activities, the daily plan can change as well. Biking uses the lower body more which can replace lower body resistance exercises, and also helps with balance. Rowing and swimming could replace upper body resistance exercises, and both can also help with balance.

Daily Reminders:

✓ Warm up and cool down for 2-5 minutes each day around exercises.

✓ Hold the stretches for 30 seconds. (If over 65 years old, then hold the stretch for 60 seconds.)

✓ Repeat each stretch at least twice and up to 4 times for each side.

✓ For resistance exercises, choose strengthening exercises that will work all the different major muscle groups. Plan a total of 8-10 exercises. Repeat each exercise 2-4 times (sets) for each side. In each set, perform 8-12 repetitions. (If over 65 years old, then perform 10-15 reps with lighter weights.)

✓ Maximum heart rate is 220 minus your age. Target heart rate during exercise is your maximum heart rate multiplied by 0.5 and by 0.85 which will give you the target range of 50-85% of your maximum heart rate. Fat burning typically happens at 60-70% maximum heart rate which is your maximum heart rate multiplied by 0.6 and 0.7 to get a range. Weight loss can occur when you reach your fat burning heart rate for at least 15 minutes.

✓ Directions of how to do the individual stretches can be found in the Flexibility Chapter.

✓ Directions for how to do the individual resistance exercises can be found in the Resistance and Strengthening Chapter.

Example Exercise Plan – Chronic Leukemia

65 year old man is receiving chemotherapy for chronic lymphocytic leukemia. It causes a little fatigue, nausea, and diarrhea. He used to be very active but has not done any regular exercise for a few years. He does still do yard work. He is going to join the local gym as they have a seniors' rate discount.

Weekly Exercise Plan – increase amount of time walking each week as stamina increases

Monday – walk 15 minutes; lower/upper body strength training; stretch lower/upper body

Tuesday –walk 15 minutes

Wednesday – walk 15 minutes; lower/upper body strengthening; stretch lower/upper body

Thursday –walk 15 minutes

Friday – walk 15 minutes; lower/upper body strengthening; stretch lower/upper body

Saturday – yard work

Sunday – walk 30 minutes

Weekly Reminders:

✓ Plan to do daily aerobic exercise daily. If he is overweight, then he should have a goal heart rate of 60-70% of his maximum heart rate for at least 15 minutes to help burn fat and maintain a normal weight. If he is not overweight, then he should have a goal heart rate of 50-85% of his maximum heart rate.

✓ Goal of 150 minutes of aerobic exercise per week but since he has not been regularly exercising and is likely deconditioned, he should start with a goal of 90 minutes and work up to a goal of 150 minutes per week.

✓ Incorporate resistance and strengthening at least 3 times per week on non-consecutive days to strengthen muscles and bones and prevent fractures. Since he is 65 years old, he should plan to do 8-10 different exercises that target all the major muscle groups, performing 10-15 repetitions of each exercise using lighter weights. (If he was under 65 years old, then he should do heavier weights or more resistance and decrease the repetitions to 8-12.) He will need to start with low amount of weight or resistance since he has not regularly done exercise.

✓ Incorporate flexibility and balance exercises, such as walking on uneven ground, 1 to 2 times per week to help prevent falls.

✓ With symptoms of nausea and diarrhea, it is important to avoid dehydration. He should try to drink 16 ounces of water an hour to two hours before any exercise, and then 8 ounces prior to exercise and about every 15 minutes during the exercise routine and again after exercise.

✓ He will be more sensitive to the sun on chemotherapy and needs to wear sunscreen when outside and long sleeve shirts and pants if not too hot. Also, he should wear gloves while doing yard work to protect his hands from injuries since chemotherapy can cause dry skin.

Daily Routine Plan

Monday, Wednesday and Friday

- walk the amount of time per week goal, goal heart rate 78-132 (50-85% maximum heart rate)
- strength training upper and lower body (using machines at the gym 10-15 reps; 2-4 sets; perform 2 sets of stretches prior to weights and 2 sets of stretches after weight machines)
  - seated chest press
  - lateral pulldowns
  - shoulder press
  - cable curls
  - press downs

- seated abs machine
- leg extension
- leg curls
- stretch upper and lower body (2 sets before weight machines and 2 sets after weight machines)
  - neck roll
  - upper shoulder stretch
  - triceps stretch
  - shoulder and chest stretch
  - hamstring stretch
  - quadriceps stretch
  - hip flexor and glute stretch
  - low back stretch

Tuesday, Thursday and Sunday
- walk the amount of time per week goal, goal heart rate 78-132 (50-85% maximum heart rate)

Saturday
- Yard work

Daily Reminders:
- ✓ Warm up and cool down for 2-5 minutes each day around exercises.
- ✓ Hold the stretches for 60 seconds. (If under 65 years old, then hold the stretch for 30 seconds.)
- ✓ Repeat each stretch at least twice and up to 4 times for each side.
- ✓ For resistance exercises, choose strengthening exercises that will work all the different major muscle groups. Plan at least 8 exercises. Repeat each exercise 2-4 times (sets) for each side.

In each set, perform 10-15 repetitions. He will need to start with low resistance or less weight since he has not been regularly exercising.

✓ Try to drink 16 ounces of water an hour to two hours before any exercise, then 8 ounces immediately prior to exercise, and about every 15 minutes during the exercise routine and again after exercise.

✓ Maximum heart rate is 220 minus your age. Target heart rate during exercise is your maximum heart rate multiplied by 0.5 and by 0.85 which will give you the target range of 50-85% of your maximum heart rate. Fat burning typically happens at 60-70% maximum heart rate which is your maximum heart rate multiplied by 0.6 and 0.7 to get a range. Weight loss can occur when you reach your fat burning heart rate for at least 15 minutes.

✓ Directions of how to do the individual stretches can be found in the Flexibility Chapter.

✓ Directions for how to do the individual strength exercises can be found in the Resistance and Strengthening Chapter.

CHAPTER 20
CAREGIVER OF A CANCER SURVIVOR

Being a caregiver for a cancer survivor can be a lot of work, but it is very rewarding. It can lead to physical and emotional exhaustion which can in turn lower the immune system, lead to health problems and financial stress. Exercise can improve the health of caregivers of cancer survivors in many the same ways that it can improve the health of a cancer survivor. In addition, it can help prevent cancer too. By improving the health of caregivers, financial savings can also occur by lowering the need for healthcare visits, tests and medicines.

There are currently about 3 million unpaid caregivers to adult cancer survivors and 30 million unpaid caregivers for varying illnesses and disabilities in the US. All caregivers, whether for cancer or other chronic illnesses and disabilities, can have similar health concerns. Research has shown that caregivers have higher levels of depression, anxiety and insomnia than the average population, and even higher levels than cancer survivors themselves. Rates of depression and anxiety in caregivers are about 50% which is twice the average population. Insomnia rates are between 50-80% in caregivers which is nearly three times the average population. This chapter will go through some of the ways exercise can help caregivers of cancer survivors by lowering stress, improving sleep, improving mood, while also providing the physical benefits of cardiovascular health and wellness. At the end of the chapter, I will outline an example work out plan for a caregiver to consider.

First, let's review the way exercise can prevent cancer. Higher rates of many types of cancer are associated with obesity, and exercise decreases obesity rates. There are also slightly higher rates of some cancers in people with diabetes, and exercise has been shown to lower the rates of diabetes and control blood sugar better in those who have diabetes. Studies have proven that those who exercise regularly have lower rates of many different cancer occurrences and recurrences. Nearly all types of exercise seem to be beneficial at lowering the rates of cancer including aerobic exercise such as walking, resistance and weight training, and yoga or stretching. Remember that the hormones produced during exercise play an important role at improving health and well-being. The hormone insulin-like growth factor which can be actually be lowered with all types of exercises, even stretching has been linked to the prevention of cancer when at lower levels. Other hormones including testosterone, growth hormone, thyroid hormone, epinephrine and insulin are involved with strengthening muscles and joints, managing the body's metabolism, and maintaining appropriate weight. Together, the hormones produced during exercise promote wellness of the body and likely all contribute to the lower rates of cancer.

Hormones can also promote wellness by lowering stress and improving mood and sleep, all of which is important to support a healthy immune system. For example, vigorous exercise increases the level of endorphins in a person's bloodstream. Endorphins are similar to morphine in molecular structure, which allows them to activate the opioid receptors in the brain and elsewhere in the body to improve that person's mood and stress in a natural way. Exercise can strengthen the muscles that support the joints putting less stress on those joints, lowering the risk of fractures, improving coordination and flexibility of the body. Better body mechanics promote health, lower the risk of falls and injuries, and improve mood. By lowering stress and anxiety, sleep is often improved as well.

It is important to incorporate into your routine all different forms of exercise which should include aerobic endurance exercises, resistance or strength training and stretching. Balance exercises can be incorporated into some of the activities to simplify your routine. The aerobic exercises should be aimed at attaining and maintaining a normal weight. Also, planning activities with the cancer survivor you are caregiving for can help motivate both of you to participate in regular exercise and provide a different way to interact with each.

Example Exercise Plan – Caregiver of a Cancer Survivor

40 year old daughter who is providing assistance to her 60 year old mom who is undergoing chemotherapy treatments for breast cancer. She has teenage children at home and she works full time but is taking some time off of work periodically to assist her mom. She previously would exercise at the gym 3-4 times per week but was not a regular daily exerciser. She has gained some weight since she has been helping with her mom and she would like to lose the weight she has gained along with a little extra. She also helps to transport her children to school and sports.

Weekly Exercise Plan

Monday – walk 20 minutes

Tuesday – walk 20 minutes; balance and resistance training; stretch upper/lower body

Wednesday – walk 20 minutes

Thursday – walk 20 minutes; balance and resistance training; stretch upper/lower body

Friday – walk 20 minutes

Saturday – walk 20 minutes; yoga class at gym

Sunday – walk 30-45 minutes; stretch upper/lower body

Weekly Reminders:

✓ Plan to do daily aerobic exercise. Goal heart rate is 60-70% of maximum heart rate for at least 15 minutes to help burn fat and maintain a normal weight.

✓ Goal of 150 minutes of moderate intensity exercise per week.

✓ Incorporate resistance and strengthening at least 2 times per week on non-consecutive days to strengthen muscles and bones and prevent fractures. Since she is under 65 years old, she should plan to do 8-10 different exercises that target all the major muscle groups, performing 8-12 repetitions of each exercise. (If she was over 65 years old, then she should do lighter weights or less resistance and increase the repetitions to 10-15.)

✓ Incorporate flexibility and balance exercises, such as yoga, 1 to 2 times per week to help prevent falls.

Daily Routine

Monday, Wednesday and Friday
- walk 20 minutes with a goal heart rate of 108-126 (60-70% maximum target heart rate)

Tuesday, Thursday
- walk 20 minutes with a goal heart rate of 108-126 (60-70% maximum target heart rate)
- resistance training using body weight exercises except biceps (8-12 reps; 2-4 sets of each;
    - 2 sets of stretches before and 2 sets of stretches after the resistance training)
    - low plank
    - push-ups
    - swimmers
    - flying
    - arm circles
    - biceps using 5 pound free weights
    - triceps dips
    - reverse crunches
    - wall sits
    - lunges (also covers balance)
- stretch upper and lower body
    - neck roll
    - upper shoulder stretch
    - triceps stretch
    - shoulder and chest stretch
    - low back/hips/hamstrings/glutes
    - hip flexors/quadriceps/back/calf (also covers balance)

Saturday

- walk 45 minutes with a friend; goal heart rate of 99-115 (60-70% maximum target heart rate)
- yoga class at the gym for strength, flexibility and balance

Sunday

- walk 30-45 minutes with a goal heart rate of 108-126 (60-70% maximum target heart rate)

Daily Reminders:

✓ Warm up and cool down for 2-5 minutes each day around exercises.

✓ Hold the stretches for 30 seconds. (If over 65 years old, then for hold for 60 seconds.)

✓ Repeat each stretch at least twice and up to 4 times for each side.

✓ For resistance exercises, chose strengthening exercises that will work all the different major muscle groups. Plan a total of 8-10 exercises. Repeat each exercise 2-4 times (sets) for each side. In each set, perform 8-12 repetitions. (If over 65 years old, then perform 10-15 reps using lighter weights.)

✓ Maximum heart rate is 220 minus your age. Target heart rate during exercise is your maximum heart rate multiplied by 0.5 and by 0.85 which will give you the target range of 50-85% of your maximum heart rate. Fat burning typically happens at 60-70% maximum heart rate which is your maximum heart rate multiplied by 0.6 and 0.7 to get a range. Weight loss can occur when you reach your fat burning heart rate for at least 15 minutes.

✓ Consider walking when waiting for a kid to finish their sports practice or during their pre-game warm-up, during a lunch break, or first thing in the morning so that it does not get put off. When feeling stronger, consider jogging in the morning a couple times a week.

✓ Directions of how to do the individual stretches can be found in the Flexibility Chapter.

✓ Directions for how to do the individual resistance exercises can be found in the Resistance and Strengthening Chapter.

CHAPTER 21
CANCER PREVENTION

Even though nearly 50% of people will be diagnosed with a cancer in their lifetime, the goal of improving health through exercise is to lower that rate to closer to 30% which is a real possibility. Since some studies have shown that regular exercise can lower the rates of cancer by as much as 35%, improving the activity levels of adults, and children, can prevent many cancers and improve survival rates. Exercise can improve the health of people without cancer in many the same ways that it can improve the health of a cancer survivor. This chapter will go through some of the ways exercise can help prevent cancer from ever occurring by lowering stress, improving sleep, improving mood, supporting a healthy immune system, while also providing the physical benefits of cardiovascular health and wellness. At the end of the chapter, I will outline an example work out plan for prevention of cancer.

Exercise has been proven to lower the risk of developing a number of different cancers, including cancers of the colon, breast, endometrium, kidney, bladder, esophagus, blood system, lung, head and neck and liver. Colon cancer is currently the second most common cancer in both women and men, occurring in about 1 in 23 people with potential rates lowered by 25% with regular exercise. This could prevent 6 out every 23 people from ever having to deal with a colon cancer diagnosis. The risk of breast cancer has been shown to be lowered by about 12% with exercise and endometrial cancer by as much as 20%. So let's consider the number of people who may be spared the ravages of cancer by regular exercise. If regular exercise can decrease the risk of a cancer by a third, and considering the average number of people who were diagnosed with cancer in 2018 was 1.7 million people, then about 560,000 people would be spared a cancer diagnosis by simply participating in regular exercise.

In addition, exercise has a financial benefit. A conservative estimate of US healthcare spending on cancer care in 2018 is 150 billion dollars which would be a cost savings of about 50 billion dollars per year if a third of cancers could be prevented with regular exercise. This could save an average person with good health insurance coverage at least $5000 out of pocket expenses per year for treatment of a cancer, not including the loss of money from inability to work. Even without a cancer diagnosis, it has been estimated that people save about $100 dollars per month in healthcare expenditure from regular exercise. This can be due to other health benefits from exercise besides cancer prevention.

Exercise can lower the rate of other health disorders such as obesity, diabetes, high cholesterol, hypertension, heart disease, and stroke. In addition, exercise can lower pain requiring less medicine and assistive devices such as braces. Exercise improves mood including depression and anxiety which can decrease the need for medicines and time off work. Regular exercise has been shown to reduce the rate of type II diabetes by about 50% which lowers the amount of treatments and other complications that could occur. Strokes can be decreased by about 25% and heart disease lowered by about 15% with regular exercise.

Nearly all types of exercise seem to be beneficial at lowering the rates of cancer including aerobic exercise such as walking, resistance and weight training, and yoga or stretching. Remember that the hormones produced during exercise play an important role at improving health and well-being. Another hormone, insulin-like growth factor, is actually lowered during exercise which can inhibit cancer cell growth and potentially prevent cancer. Other hormones including testosterone, growth hormone, thyroid hormone, epinephrine and insulin are involved with strengthening muscles and joints, managing the body's metabolism, and maintaining appropriate weight. Together, the hormones produced during exercise promote wellness of the body and likely all contribute to the lower rates of cancer.

Hormones also promote wellness that help lower stress and improve mood and sleep, all of which is important to support a healthy immune system. Endorphins, which are increased in the blood of people who participate in vigorous exercise, are structurally similar to morphine and can activate opioid receptors in the brain and elsewhere to improve mood and stress. Exercise can strengthen the muscles that support the joints putting less stress on those joints, lowering the risk of fractures, improving coordination and flexibility of the body. Better body mechanics promote health, lower the risk of falls and injuries, and improve mood. By lowering stress and anxiety, sleep is often improved as well.

It is important to incorporate into your routine all different forms of exercise which should include aerobic endurance exercises, resistance or strength training and stretching. Balance exercises can be incorporated into some of the activities to simplify your routine. The aerobic exercises should be aimed at attaining and maintaining a normal weight.

Example Exercise Plan – Preventing Cancer

35 year old woman whose father recently was diagnosed with colon cancer at the age of 65 and he required surgery and chemotherapy. She wants to do everything possible to lower her risk of developing cancer. She is married, works full time and has 1 child, age 7. She exercises off and on but not regularly. She does belong to a gym but has difficulty finding the time to go. She would like to lose about 10 pounds.

Weekly Exercise Plan – first 2 months

Monday – walk 20-30 minutes in morning

Tuesday – Gym – work with trainer to develop arm and leg strengthening exercise program including stretching OR do weights at home

Wednesday – walk 20-30 minutes in morning

Thursday – Gym – work with trainer to develop arm and leg strengthening exercise program including stretching OR do weights at home

Friday – walk 20-30 minutes in morning

Saturday – yoga class at gym

Sunday – walk 30-45 minutes; stretch upper and lower body

Weekly Plan – month 2 onward

Monday – jog 30 minutes in morning

Tuesday – Gym arm/leg strengthening exercise program including stretching OR home weights

Wednesday – jog 30 minutes in morning

Thursday – Gym arm/leg strengthening exercise program including stretching OR home weights

Friday – jog 30 minutes in morning

Saturday – yoga class at gym

Sunday – walk 60 minutes; stretch upper and lower body

Weekly Reminders:

✓ Plan to do daily aerobic exercise. Goal heart rate is 60-70% of maximum heart rate for at least 15 minutes to help burn fat and maintain a normal weight.

✓ Goal of 150 minutes of moderate intensity exercise per week.

✓ Incorporate resistance and strengthening at least 2 times per week on non-consecutive days to strengthen muscles and bones and prevent fractures. Since she is under 65 years old, she should plan to do 8-10 different exercises that target all the major muscle groups, performing 8-12 repetitions of each exercise. (If she was over 65 years old, then she should do lighter weights or less resistance and increase the repetitions to 10-15.)

✓ Incorporate flexibility and balance exercises, such as yoga, 1 to 2 times per week to help prevent falls.

Daily Routine – first 2 months

Monday, Wednesday and Friday
- walk 20 – 30 minutes with a goal heart rate of 111-130 (60-70% maximum target heart rate)

Tuesday and Thursday
- Gym arm and leg strengthening with trainer (8-12 reps; 2-4 sets of each) with stretching (2 sets
    - of stretches before and 2 sets of stretches training)
- OR weights at home
    - low plank – no weights
    - push-ups – no weights
    - arm circles – 2 pound weight
    - biceps – 5 pound free weights
    - kickbacks for triceps – 2 pound weights
    - reverse crunches – no weights
    - wall sits – 15-30 seconds
    - lunges (also covers balance) – 2 pound weights
- stretch upper and lower body
    - neck roll
    - upper shoulder stretch
    - triceps stretch
    - shoulder and chest stretch
    - low back/hips/hamstrings/glutes
    - hip flexors/quadriceps/back/calf (also covers balance)

Saturday
- yoga class at the gym for strength, flexibility and balance

Sunday

- walk 30-45 minutes with a goal heart rate of 111-130 (60-70% maximum target heart rate)

Daily Routine – month 2 onward

Monday, Wednesday and Friday
- jog 30 minutes with a goal heart rate of 111-130 (60-70% maximum target heart rate)

Tuesday and Thursday
- Gym arm and leg strengthening (8-12 reps; 2-4 sets of each) with stretching (2 sets
    - of stretches before and 2 sets of stretches training)
- OR weights at home
    - low plank – no weights
    - push-ups – no weights
    - arm circles – 5 pound weight
    - biceps – 8 pound free weights
    - kickbacks for triceps – 5 pound weights
    - reverse crunches – no weights
    - wall sits – 45-60 seconds
    - lunges (also covers balance) – 5 pound weights
- stretch upper and lower body
    - neck roll
    - upper shoulder stretch
    - triceps stretch
    - shoulder and chest stretch
    - low back/hips/hamstrings/glutes
    - hip flexors/quadriceps/back/calf (also covers balance)

Saturday
- yoga class at the gym for strength, flexibility and balance

Sunday

- walk 60 minutes with a goal heart rate of 111-130 (60-70% maximum target heart rate)

Daily Reminders:

- ✓ Warm up and cool down for 2-5 minutes each day around exercises.
- ✓ Hold the stretches for 30 seconds. (If over 65 years old, then for hold for 60 seconds.)
- ✓ Repeat each stretch at least twice and up to 4 times for each side.
- ✓ For resistance exercises, chose strengthening exercises that will work all the different major muscle groups. Plan a total of 8-10 exercises. Repeat each exercise 2-4 times (sets) for each side. In each set, perform 8-12 repetitions. (If over 65 years old, then perform 10-15 reps using lighter weights.)
- ✓ Maximum heart rate is 220 minus your age. Target heart rate during exercise is your maximum heart rate multiplied by 0.5 and by 0.85 which will give you the target range of 50-85% of your maximum heart rate. Fat burning typically happens at 60-70% maximum heart rate which is your maximum heart rate multiplied by 0.6 and 0.7 to get a range. Weight loss can occur when you reach your fat burning heart rate for at least 15 minutes.
- ✓ Consider walking with a friend to keep the motivation up. Or consider changing the walking time to during the kid's sports practices or other kid's group activity time.
- ✓ Directions of how to do the individual stretches can be found in the Flexibility Chapter.
- ✓ Directions for how to do the individual resistance exercises can be found in the Resistance and Strengthening Chapter.

SECTION 5
PERSONAL JOURNAL

CHAPTER 22
MONTHLY PLANNING

To have a successful exercise plan, you should plan your monthly calendar in advance. When you plan your month in advance, you set expectations for yourself which helps with the success. Also, it helps you look at time constraints that occur in your personal or work life that may alter how you are able to exercise. By preparing in advance, you can make sure there is time to get all your planned exercises completed. As you put together your exercise plan, here is a list of things to remember that have been previously discussed in this book.

- If you are over the age of 20 years old, your goal should be at least 30 minutes per day of exercise. This can be split up into smaller increments.
- You need a combination of aerobic/endurance, balance, flexibility, and resistance/strengthening. Some of these exercises can be combined for an efficient work out.
- Adults goal for aerobic or endurance exercise is at least 150 minutes of moderate intensity exercise, or 75 minutes of vigorous intensity exercise each week, preferably spread throughout the week.
- Try to incorporate moderate activity such as brisk walking on at least 3 of the days per week.
- Getting your heart rate up to 60-70% of your target heart rate will help burn fat, and reaching this target heart rate for at least 15 minutes will help you lose weight if this is a goal.

- You should try to do resistance and strengthening at least 2 times per week on non-consecutive days. Plan to do 8-10 different exercises that target all the major muscle groups. For people under 65 year old, do 8-12 repetitions of each exercise and for people over 65 years old, do lighter weights or less resistance and increase the repetitions to 10-15.

- Reminder about how to calculate heart rate goal for fat burning which occurs at 60-70% of your target heart rate. First calculate your maximum heart rate by subtracting your age from 220. For instance, a 50 year old will have a maximum heart rate of 170 bpm. Then calculate your target heart rate during exercise by multiplying your maximum heart rate by 0.5 and by 0.85 which will give you the target range of 50-85% of your maximum heart rate. So a 50 year old will have a target heart rate range of 85-145 bpm during exercise which is 50-85% of their maximum heart rate. Fat burning typically happens at 60-70% maximum heart rate. So for a 50 year old, multiply the maximum heart rate of 170 bpm by 0.6 and 0.7 to give you the target fat burning range which is 102-119 bpm. Usually you will need to reach 60-70% of your maximum heart rate for at least 15 minutes to lose weight.

Example

Weekly Plan for a 50 year old woman who wants to lose a little weight (goal fat burning occurs at 60-70% of the maximum heart rate which for this 50 year old is 102-119 bpm)

Monday	Yoga
Tuesday	Walk 30 minutes (heart rate goal 102-119)
Wednesday	Resistance bands 45 minutes
Thursday	Walk 30 minutes (heart rate goal 102-119)
Friday	Resistance bands 45 minutes
Saturday	Walk 60 minutes (heart rate goal 102-119)
Sunday	Walk 30 minutes (heart rate goal 102-119)

My Weekly Plan

Aerobic exercise goal per week (minutes):
Stretching goals per week (days):

Resistance or Strength Training per week (days):
Balance Training per week (days):

Monday:

Tuesday:

Wednesday:

Thursday:

Friday:

Saturday:

Sunday:

My Weekly Plan

Aerobic exercise goal per week (minutes):
Stretching goals per week (days):

Resistance or Strength Training per week (days):
Balance Training per week (days):

Monday:

Tuesday:

Wednesday:

Thursday:

Friday:

Saturday:

Sunday:

My Weekly Plan

Aerobic exercise goal per week (minutes):
Stretching goals per week (days):

Resistance or Strength Training per week (days):
Balance Training per week (days):

Monday:

Tuesday:

Wednesday:

Thursday:

Friday:

Saturday:

Sunday:

CHAPTER 23
DAILY JOURNAL

Planning a daily exercise journal can help make sure your exercise routine each day is well-balanced with all the different activities you need to stay healthy. Looking back over time at your successes can help you prepare new goals when you are ready. Keeping track of the number of reps and amount of weight you use in your exercise routine can help you increase your weights and sets appropriately and safely to avoid injuries. Also, it keeps you from forgetting to do something. Here are some things to remember as you develop your daily plan.

- If you are over the age of 20 years old, your goal should be at least 30 minutes per day of exercise. This can be broken down into smaller incremen ts for success.
- Warm up for 2-3 minutes prior to starting an activity to prevent injury.
- Cool down for 5-10 minutes after an activity to also prevent injury and help your muscles recover. This is a good time to incorporate stretching and deep breathing exercises.
- When stretching, remember that if you are under 65 years of age, it is recommended to hold each stretch for a count of 30 seconds, with a 10 second rest after the stretch before repeating. For those over 65 years of age, it is recommended to hold the stretch for 60 seconds for maximum benefit with a 10 second rest after the stretch.

- When doing your aerobic exercises, your goal target heart rate is 50-85% of your maximum heart rate which is 220 minus your age in years. You can maximize fat burning by having your target heart rate at 60-70% of your maximum heart rate. If you keep it there for 15 minutes, you can start losing weight if this is a goal.

- Reminder about how to calculate heart rate goal for fat burning which occurs at 60-70% of your target heart rate. First calculate your maximum heart rate by subtracting your age from 220. For instance, a 50 year old will have a maximum heart rate of 170 bpm. Then calculate your target heart rate during exercise by multiplying your maximum heart rate by 0.5 and by 0.85 which will give you the target range of 50-85% of your maximum heart rate. So a 50 year old will have a target heart rate range of 85-145 bpm during exercise which is 50-85% of their target heart rate. Fat burning typically happens at 60-70% maximum heart rate. So for a 50 year old, multiply the maximum heart rate of 170 bpm by 0.6 and 0.7 to give you the target fat burning range which is 102-119 bpm. Usually you will need to reach 60-70% of your maximum heart rate for at least 15 minutes to lose weight.

Example of a Daily Journal for a 50 year old man who wants to lose a little weight (goal heart rate for fat burning is 60-70% of your maximum heart rate range for at least 15 minutes which would be 102-119 bpm for an average 50 year old man)

Daily Routine

Monday

- Tai Chi: Tai Chi video for 30 minutes of Tai Chi. This will include flexibility stretches, balance, and strength exercises using body resistance.

Tuesday and Thursday

- Walk: Warm up 2-3 minutes with a slower walk. Then walk for 30 minutes
- Stretches for cool down for 10 minutes
  - neck rolls
  - triceps stretch
  - shoulder and chest stretch
  - low back/hips/hamstrings/glutes stretch
  - low back/hips/obliques/glutes/quadriceps stretch

Wednesday and Friday

- Warm up for 2-3 minutes with some marching in place and 20 jumping jacks
- Resistance exercises:
  - 2 planks holding for 30 seconds each
  - 2 sets of 10 standard push-ups
  - 2 sets of chair dips (8-10 reps each set)
  - 2 sets of standing bicep curls with a band (10 reps each arm/set)

- 2 sets of triceps kickbacks with a band (10 reps each arm/set)
- 2 sets of squats without a band (10 reps each set)
- 2 sets of lunges without a band (10 reps each leg/set)
- 2 sets of hip raises (20 reps each set)
- 2 sets of crunches (10 reps each set)
- 2 sets of standing sit-ups (20 reps each set)
- 2 sets of trunk rotations with a band (10 reps each set)

- Cool down stretches for 10 minutes
  - neck rolls
  - triceps stretch
  - shoulder and chest stretch
  - low back/hips/hamstrings/glutes stretch
  - low back/hips/obliques/glutes/quadriceps stretch

Saturday and Sunday
- Walk – Warm up 2-3 minutes and then walk for 30-50 minutes.
- Stretches for cool down for 10 minutes
  - neck rolls
  - triceps stretch
  - shoulder and chest stretch
  - low back/hips/hamstrings/glutes stretch
  - low back/hips/obliques/glutes/quadriceps stretch

My Daily Plan

Monday:

Tuesday:

Wednesday:

Thursday:

Friday:

Saturday:

Sunday:

My Daily Plan

Day of Week

Exercise

Goals: Heart Rate/Time

My Daily Plan

Exercise

Day of Week

Goals: Heart Rate/Time